CALCULATION SKILLS
FOR NURSES

Student Survival Skills Series

Survive your nursing course with these essential guides for all student nurses:

Calculation Skills for Nurses
Claire Boyd
9781118448892

Medicine Management Skills for Nurses
Claire Boyd
9781118448854

Clinical Skills for Nurses
Claire Boyd
9781118448779

CALCULATION SKILLS
FOR NURSES

Claire Boyd
RGN, Cert Ed
Practice Development Trainer

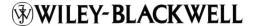

A John Wiley & Sons, Ltd., Publication

Registered office:
John Wiley & Sons, Ltd, The Atrium, Southern Gate, Chichester, West Sussex, PO19 8SQ, UK

Editorial offices:
9600 Garsington Road, Oxford, OX4 2DQ, UK
The Atrium, Southern Gate, Chichester, West Sussex, PO19 8SQ, UK
111 River Street, Hoboken, NJ 07030-5774, USA

For details of our global editorial offices, for customer services and for information about how to apply for permission to reuse the copyright material in this book please see our website at www.wiley.com/wiley-blackwell.

Library of Congress Cataloging-in-Publication Data
Boyd, Claire.
 Calculation skills for nurses / Claire Boyd, RGN, cert. ed., practice development trainer.
    pages cm. – (Student survival skills series)
 Includes bibliographical references and index.
 ISBN 978-1-118-44889-2 (pbk. : alk. paper) – ISBN 978-1-118-44891-5 (epub) – ISBN 978-1-118-44893-9 (mobi) – ISBN 978-1-118-44895-3 (epdf/ebook) 1. Nursing–Mathematics. 2. Pharmaceutical arithmetic. I. Title.
 RT68.B67 2013
 615.1'401513–dc23

                                                                                    2012039434

A catalogue record for this book is available from the British Library.

Cover image courtesy of Visual Philosophy
Cover design by Visual Philosophy
Part title/chapter opener image courtesy of iStockphoto

Set in Trade Gothic Light 9/12pt by Aptara Inc., New Delhi, India
Printed and bound in Malaysia by Vivar Printing Sdn Bhd

1 2013

Contents

Part 3: Putting It All Into Practice 97

Part 4: Testing Your Knowledge 143

Part 5: Appendices 163

Preface

This book is designed to assist student healthcare workers in the field of calculations. All exercises are related to practice and the healthcare environment. Chapter 1 takes the student through the basics, with Chapter 2 incorporating a pre-assessment quiz to identify any areas needing to be revisited (referring the reader back to specific sections in Chapter 1). The book then goes through the 'bread and butter' of everyday calculations used on a daily basis in health care.

The book incorporates many activities to check understanding, and is laid out in a simple to follow step-by-step approach. It ends with four Knowledge tests that relate everything the reader has learned to practice situations. The book also incorporates an example of an Employment Services calculations test paper, as students are often asked to complete a calculations test when being interviewed for a job. All answers can be located at the back of the book.

The aim of this book is to start the individual on a journey through many healthcare-related exercises in order to build confidence and competence. It has been compiled using quotes and tips from student nurses themselves; it is a book by students for students.

Claire Boyd
Bristol
October 2012

Introduction

Hello, my name is Claire.

Working as a Practice Development Trainer for a large NHS trust, it was with sadness that I came across experienced, competent nurses who were paralysed with fear while sitting their calculations test (a prerequisite for being able to attend the Intravenous (IV) Study day in my trust, and administer IV drugs, including IV fluids). Many NHS trusts follow this maxim. Fifty per cent of those sitting the IV test were referred, not necessarily through incompetence, but more likely through a fear of maths. Combine this with a fear of exams and we have a recipe for failure.

Since instigating Calculations Master Classes and, for those too embarrassed or shy, individual tuition, the pass rate has risen to 98% on first attempts. This proved that with a little nurturing, a sprinkling of fun and a dollop of blood, sweat and tears we could all pass this test. Fear of maths was the biggest hurdle and once removed, these nurses were flying! Many of the nurses coming to see me explained how they had had bad experiences since school and how many had compensated by avoiding anything to do with solving difficult maths problems in their clinical areas. This is quite amazing because in the healthcare profession maths confronts us on a daily basis, be it converting a patient's weight from stones to kilograms, totting up fluid charts or dispensing tablets and capsules. Difficulty with maths is not peculiar to the health profession: the Moser Report (DfEE, 1999) suggested that as many as 40% of UK adults have some numeracy problems. The problem in nursing is that if *we* make a calculations error we could seriously harm our patients, or even worse.

Trained nurses or student nurses, why is it that we always feel that everyone else is a maths genius and we alone are struggling? Even old Einstein struggled with his maths, and he was a genius! I have not yet met a nurse who is incapable of passing a calculations test in preparation for administering IV drugs. First, remove the fear factor. Second, add some humour. Third, break down each question and 'see' what is required to solve the problem. Start with the basics and from this we can build up to more complicated problems, and support our colleagues in the workplace, helping them to gain competence and confidence.

I was asked to include student nurses in the Calculations Master Classes and thus our working relationship was forged. It was by listening to their comments – their wants and needs – that this book came to fruition. The book has four parts. Part 1 tests your ability and gives you pointers for revision. Part 2 gets to grips with the basics that you will meet in the healthcare environment. Part 3 puts the basics into practice and shows how the calculations you have learned may be applied. Part 4 then lets you test everything you have learned.

The book aims to relate practice to theory. What is the point of using examples in a healthcare-orientated calculations book that talk about the cost of a bag of sugar, or how many people are getting on and off a train in certain stations (unless, of course, they are going to work in a healthcare setting)! Let's make it specific and relevant.

I believe firmly in using formulas for working out drug dosages, but I am aware that an understanding of how these formulas work must first be established, and a rough estimate of the correct answer should always be at the back of our minds. It is also with this principle that we need to start with the basics, to gain understanding, and from this we can build up to more complicated problems. It is for this reason I have produced the formulas in a handy format on the inside back cover for you to photocopy and laminate (for infection control, to be wiped clean) and keep in your pocket. No more writing these out on tongue decompressors: we've all seen it!

In short, this book is designed to instil confidence and competence in the area of calculations to the student nurse, assistant practitioner, operating department practitioner, newly qualified nurse and anyone else requiring assistance in this field. It is designed to be used as a building block, a platform for the rest of your healthcare career. There is a heavy emphasis on conversions, as changing the dose prescribed on a prescription chart, which may be written in grams, to correspond with the format on the ampoule, which may be written in milligrams, is one of the fundamental skills in which we need to be competent from the outset.

Throughout the book you will come across the Quick Tips feature, which will give you gems, quotes and advice from real student nurses who have trodden the same path that you are now taking.

So, grab a pen, paper and calculator (if you wish to use one). Put on some music or move to a quiet space (if this is how you like to study), make a cup of tea or pour a glass of water (or whatever you fancy), pick up some digestive biscuits, and settle down to some calculations.

First, let's have some fun with numbers. Use a calculator if you wish. I will tell you your age. Do you believe me?

- Multiply the first number of your age by 5 (for example, if you are 21 years of age = 2 × 5, if you are 40 years old = 4 × 5).

- Add 3 to the result.

- Double your answer.

- Add the second digit of your age to this number (for example, if you are 21, add 1, if you are 40, add 0).

- Subtract 6 from your answer.

The answer you have is your age! Clever or what?

OK, so this is a maths trick that anyone can do, but I just wanted to show you that maths can be fun and let's start removing the fear factor.

Reference
Department of Education (1999) *The Moser Report*. HMSO, London.

Acknowledgements

I, along with the publishers, would particularly like to thank all the students who helped develop this book into what it is. In particular Carla Mosser, Sami-Jo Joyce, Claire Bishop and Roxanne Barrington, and all the nursing students from the University of the West of England for the use of their tips and quotes.

Acknowledgements also go to North Bristol NHS Trust: Jane Hadfield (Head of Learning and Development) and Dr Karen Mead (Specialist Practitioner of Transfusion for NBT). Thanks also go to the NBT Library Staff for their assistance.

Special thanks also go to North Bristol NHS Trust for allowing the reproduction of the Bristol Observation Chart and drug prescription chart.

I would also like to extend my thanks to Magenta Styles (Executive Editor) for her guidance and direction and to Catriona Cooper (Project Editor), both at Wiley-Blackwell.

I dedicate this book to my loving family: husband Rob (for the use of his photographs), and Simon, Louise and David for all their assistance in helping to develop this book.

Latin Abbreviations

Here is a list of some Latin abbreviations that you may see on prescription forms.

AC   *ante cibum* (before food)

BD   *bis die* (twice daily)

OD   *omni die* (every day)

OM   *omni mane* (every morning)

ON   *omni nocte* (every night)

PC   *post cibum* (after food)

PRN   *pro re nata* (when required)

QDS   *quater die sumendus* (to be taken four times daily)

QQH   *quarta quaque hora* (every 4 hours)

STAT   immediately

TDS   *ter die sumendus* (to be taken three times daily)

TID   *ter in die* (three times daily)

The 24-Hour Clock

Time	24-hour clock
1 am	01:00
2 am	02:00
3 am	03:00
4 am	04:00
5 am	05:00
6 am	06:00
7 am	07:00
8 am	08:00
9 am	09:00
10 am	10:00
11 am	11:00
12 midday	12:00
1 pm	13:00
2 pm	14:00
3 pm	15:00
4 pm	16:00
5 pm	17:00
6 pm	18:00
7 pm	19:00
8 pm	20:00
9 pm	21:00
10 pm	22:00
11 pm	23:00
12 midnight	24:00

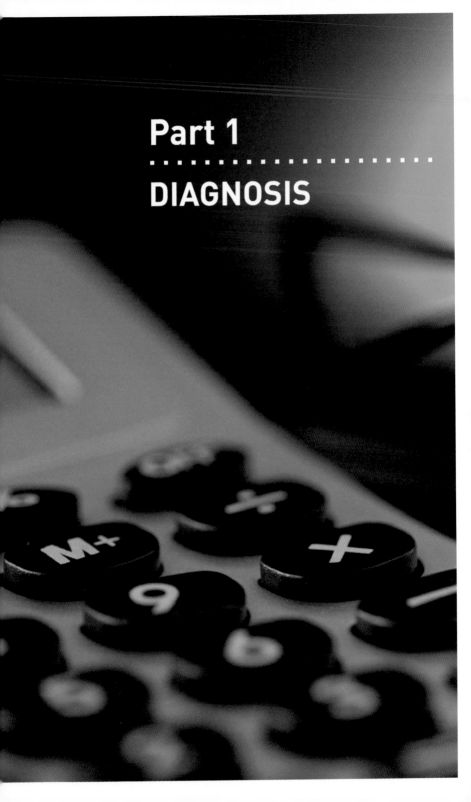

Part 1

DIAGNOSIS

Chapter 1
....
CALCULATIONS REVISION

Calculation Skills for Nurses, First Edition. Claire Boyd
© 2013 John Wiley & Sons, Ltd. Published 2013 by John Wiley & Sons Ltd.

LEARNING OUTCOMES

By the end of this chapter you will have familiarised yourself with the basics of decimals, metric measures, percentages, fractions, ratios and averages.

FEELING A BIT RUSTY?

Don't worry if picking up this book and the word 'calculations' gave you palpitations! We'll start nice and gently and summarise the basics. You may remember most of this already and feel confident enough to skip the chapter completely, and go straight to the self-assessment test in Chapter 2, or you may need to build up your confidence and reacquaint yourself with the basics.

Symbols and Signs

+	plus or addition sign; example: **6 + 9 = 15**
−	decrease, subtract or minus sign; example: **11 − 4 = 7**
×	multiply or 'times by' sign; example: **9 × 6 = 54**
÷ or **/**	division or 'divide by' sign; example: **25/5 = 5**
=	the equals sign; example: **9 × 10 = 90**
:	ratio
>	greater than
<	less than

Seeing this sign **/** means divided by…

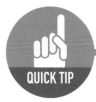

QUICK TIP

It is a good idea to reacquaint yourself with your times tables.

×	1	2	3	4	5	6	7	8	9	10	11	12
1	1	2	3	4	5	6	7	8	9	10	11	12
2	2	4	6	8	10	12	14	16	18	20	22	24
3	3	6	9	12	15	18	21	24	27	30	33	36
4	4	8	12	16	20	24	28	32	36	40	44	48
5	5	10	15	20	25	30	35	40	45	50	55	60
6	6	12	18	24	30	36	42	48	54	60	66	72
7	7	14	21	28	35	42	49	56	63	70	77	84
8	8	16	24	32	40	48	56	64	72	80	88	96
9	9	18	27	36	45	54	63	72	81	90	99	108
10	10	20	30	40	50	60	70	80	90	100	110	120
11	11	22	33	44	55	66	77	88	99	110	121	132
12	12	24	36	48	60	72	84	96	108	120	132	144

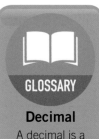

GLOSSARY

Decimal

A decimal is a number that is expressed in the counting system that uses units of tens.

DECIMAL

Decimal numbers describe tenths, hundredths and thousandths of a number. For example, 1.25 is equal to one whole unit, plus a fraction of one (25 hundredths).

Rounding Decimal Numbers

Sometimes it is necessary to 'round up' or 'round down' a decimal number or a whole number. This is particularly true in infusion drip rate calculations, as it is impossible to give a 'point' or part of a drop when setting an infusion rate; for example, 7.2 drops: how would you get the 0.2? Other medication calculations may need to be highly accurate and *incorporate* all the 'points', but as a general rule:

If the number after the point is 4 or less: round down
If the number after the point is 5 or more: round up

This is often known as the 'rule of 5s'.
Therefore, 7.2 drops becomes 7 drops only; 2.8 becomes 3.

QUICK TIP

I get it! Decimal places are numbers to the right of the decimal point. Example: 5.72 has two decimal places.

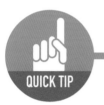

Let me show you an example...

e.g.

EXAMPLE

39.4 rounds down to **39**
2.82 rounds down to **2.8** (one decimal place)
0.864 rounds down to **0.86** (two decimal places)
31.7 rounds up to **32**
39.8 rounds up to **40**
1.65 rounds up to **1.7** (one decimal place)
0.421 rounds down to **0.42** (two decimal places)

Now, have a go at working some out for yourself: You didn't really expect me to do all the work, did you?

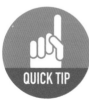

QUICK TIP

Add a zero before the decimal point: for example, .2 should be 0.2, otherwise it could be mistaken for 2.

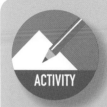

Activity 1.1

ACTIVITY

Round each of the following to one decimal place.

SECTION ONE
1   2.66
2   1.32
3   1.75
4   1.98
5   4.64

Round each of the following to the nearest whole number.

SECTION TWO
1   55.8
2   43.2
3   99.56
4   33.33
5   66.66

METRIC MEASURES

The metric system is based on multiples of 10.
So, for weight:

1 kilogram (kg)	=	1000 grams (g)
1 gram (g)	=	1000 milligrams (mg)
1 milligram (mg)	=	1000 micrograms
1 microgram	=	1000 nanograms (ng)
1 nanogram (ng)	=	1000 picograms (pg)

NOTE: where medications are concerned micrograms should *not* be abbreviated on prescription charts to mcg. This is due to the abbreviations for milligram (mg) and microgram (mcg) being quite similar, and they may be mis-read by the person administering the drug. As a nurse you may also see μ, which is another way of writing 'micro'. So, μg means micrograms.

Nanograms and picograms are very small units indeed (and are very rarely used in prescriptions).

For volume:

1 litre (L) = 1000 millilitres (mL)

Conversion from One Unit to Another

In drug calculations it is best to work in whole numbers – that is, 125 micrograms and not 0.125 mg – as fewer mistakes may be made. Therefore it is necessary to be able to convert easily from one unit to another. To do this you have to multiply or divide by a thousand.

Converting Larger Units to the Next Smaller Unit

To convert a larger unit to a smaller unit you multiply by 1000.

NOTE: the × symbol means multiply.

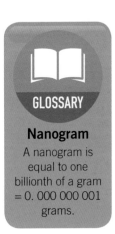

GLOSSARY

Nanogram

A nanogram is equal to one billionth of a gram = 0. 000 000 001 grams.

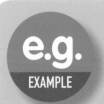

Let me show you an example...

Convert 5 g to milligrams: $5 \times 1000 = 5000$ mg
Convert 0.25 kg to grams: $0.25 \times 1000 = 250$ g
This can be done another way, simply by 'bouncing' the decimal point.
To multiply by 1000 you move the decimal point three places to the right.

Changing 5 g to milligrams: 5 . 0 0 0 g   = 5000 mg

Converting Smaller Units to the Next Larger Unit

To convert a smaller unit to the next larger unit you divide by 1000.

NOTE: the / symbol = Divided by.

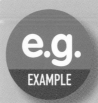

Let me show you an example...

Convert 6000 g to kilograms: 6000/1000 = 6 kg

Convert 325 mg to grams: 325/1000 = 0.325 g

To bounce using the decimal point method.

To divide by 1000 you move the decimal point three places to the left.

Changing 5000 mg to grams: 5000.0 mg = 5 g

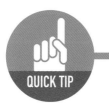

Once you have written a decimal point in your result, any noughts at the end of the answer become unnecessary.

For example: 0.6000 is written as 0.6.

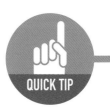

Here is a quick way of remembering this: going up to larger units: divide and move decimal place to the left ↑ ÷ ← ·

going down to smaller units: multiply and move decimal place to the right ↓ × · →

9

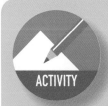

Activity 1.2

SECTION ONE

1 6000 mg to grams
2 39 000 mL to litres
3 350 mL to litres
4 0.07 micrograms to milligrams
5 4000 g to kilograms
6 4500 mg to grams
7 0.8 mg to micrograms
8 9 micrograms to nanograms
9 1300 g to kilograms
10 0.462 mg to grams

SECTION TWO

1 0.72 g to mg
2 1.4 mg to micrograms
3 0.03 g to milligrams
4 2 g to kilograms
5 2.5 L to millilitres
6 0.7 mg to micrograms
7 61.25 L to millilitres
8 92 kg to grams
9 0.02 mg to micrograms
10 0.023 mg to grams

SECTION THREE

1 20 micrograms to mg
2 634 g to kilograms
3 0.0635 mg to micrograms
4 0.25 micrograms to nanograms
5 8 kg to grams
6 1527 micrograms to milligrams
7 21.9 L to millilitres
8 64.5 micrograms to milligrams
9 349.8 g to kilograms
10 50 mL to litres

SECTION FOUR

1 3 L to millilitres
2 1.2 mg to micrograms
3 0.04 mg to micrograms
4 0.12 g to milligrams
5 0.02 mg to grams
6 0.02 micrograms to nanograms
7 2.386 kg to grams
8 4 ng to micrograms
9 1234 mL to litres
10 320 mg to grams

PERCENTAGES

Fractions, decimals and percentages all represent parts of a whole. For example:

50% = 0.5 = ½ = one half

A bag of 5% glucose means that there are 5 parts of glucose per 100 parts of water. 'Per cent' means 'per 100'.

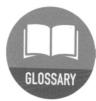

Percentage
A percentage is a way of expressing a number as a fraction of 100.

GLOSSARY

Calculating the Percentage of a Number

$$\text{Value} = \frac{\text{number}}{100} \times \text{percentage required}$$

Let me show you an example...

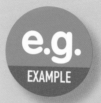

EXAMPLE

Mrs Noto has to decrease her 160 mL of medication by 15%. How many millilitres has this to be reduced by? In other words, how much of the medication does Mrs Noto still have to take?

$$\frac{160}{100} \times 15 = \frac{8}{5} \times 15 = 24 \text{ mL}$$

$$160 \text{ mL minus } 24 \text{ mL} = 136 \text{ mL}$$

Mrs Noto still needs to take 136 mL of the medication.

Finding One Amount as a Percentage of Another

$$\text{Percentage} = \frac{\text{smaller number}}{\text{larger number}} \times 100$$

Let me show you an example...

e.g.
EXAMPLE

In a calculations test 280 student nurses out of 400 passed the test first time. What percentage was this?

$$\frac{280}{400} \times 100 = \frac{280}{4} = 70\%$$

Now have a go at working some examples out for yourself.

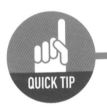

Remember: a percentage indicates a number of parts in a hundred.

QUICK TIP

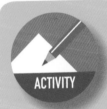

Activity 1.3

ACTIVITY

Calculate the following:
1 20% of 450 mL
2 15% of 1200 mL
3 In a numeracy test 240 out of 300 score more than 50. What percentage is this?
4 In a Clinical Directorate 85 out of 400 nursing staff are male. What percentage is this?

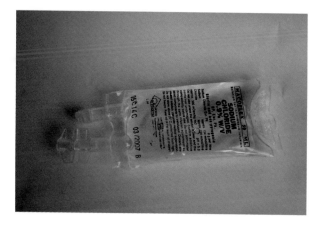

NOTE: did you ever wonder how much 0.9% sodium chloride in grams there is in 1 L of fluid? This is known as weight in volume, or w/v. We work this out:

$$\frac{0.9\%}{100} \times 1000 \text{ mL} = 9 \text{ g}$$

In a 50 mL bag of fluid, this would equate to 0.45 g (or 450 mg).

$$\frac{0.9\%}{100} \times 50 \text{ mL} = 0.45 \text{ g}$$

NOTE: percentage concentrations can be expressed in the following ways:

w/w	weight in weight
w/v	weight in volume
v/v	volume in volume

Strength of a Solution

This can be expressed as percentage weight versus volume = number of grams per 100 mL. For example, 30% sodium chloride = 30 grams in 100 mL.

Some drugs, such as local anaesthetics, are also presented in solutions of different percentages. To work out how many milligrams per millilitre there are in 1% lignocaine, we already know that 1% means 1 in 100.

Convention tells us that 1 mL is equivalent to 1 g. Therefore, 1% lignocaine means that there is 1 g of anaesthetic in every 100 mL of the solution. We could also say that there are 1000 mg of lignocaine in 100 mL of solution.

1 mL of 1% lignocaine will therefore contain:

$$\frac{1000}{100} = 10 \text{ mg/mL}$$

Therefore, 1% of lignocaine is equivalent to 10 mg per mL.

FRACTIONS

Many drug calculations require you to work with fractions. A fraction is a portion of a whole that indicates division into equal parts. For example: one large tablet cut into quarters:

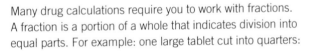

$$\frac{1 \text{ large tablet}}{4} = \frac{1}{4}$$

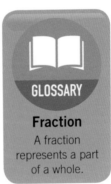

GLOSSARY

Fraction
A fraction represents a part of a whole.

NOTE: when administering medications, tablets should only ever be cut into halves, if the tablet is scored (has a line down its centre). Tablets should *never* be broken into four pieces as this is too inaccurate a dose.

Simplifying Fractions

To cancel down (or simplify) a fraction, you will need to divide the numerator and the denominator by the same number. This is called a common factor.

Example 1:

$$\frac{25}{55} = \frac{5}{11} \text{ Common factor} = 5$$

Example 2:

$$\frac{100}{225} = \frac{4}{9} \text{ Common factor} = 25$$

NOTE:

$$\frac{2}{4} = \frac{3}{6} = \frac{4}{8} = \frac{5}{10}$$

These are all the same as $\frac{1}{2}$, or, expressed another way, 50%.

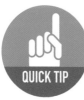

QUICK TIP

The numerator is the top number in a fraction and a denominator is the bottom number.

Changing Fractions into Decimals

Divide the top number by the bottom number.

Example:

$$\frac{4}{5} = 4.0 \text{ divided by } 5 = 0.8$$

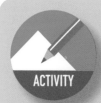

ACTIVITY

Activity 1.4

Change the following fractions to decimals, giving your answer to one decimal place.

1 $\frac{25}{3}$ **2** $\frac{15}{2}$ **3** $\frac{175}{5}$ **4** $\frac{125}{6}$ **5** $\frac{250}{6}$ **6** $\frac{122}{7}$

Simple Conversions from Fractions, Decimals and Percentages

Let me show you something:

$$\frac{20}{100} \text{ can be broken down to } \frac{2}{10}$$

by removing one zero from the top and one from the bottom.

This can be broken down to '2 goes into 2 once, and 2 goes into 10 five times'. This makes a *simplified fraction*:

$$\frac{1}{5}$$

This is the same as 20%: 20% is one-fifth of 100%, as there are five lots of 20 in 100%.

Fraction	Simplified fraction	How this is expressed in words	Decimals	Percentage
$\frac{10}{100}$	$\frac{1}{10}$	One-tenth	0.1 (0.10)	10%
$\frac{20}{100}$	$\frac{1}{5}$	One-fifth	0.2 (0.20)	20%
$\frac{25}{100}$	$\frac{1}{4}$	One-quarter	0.25	25%
$\frac{33}{100}$	$\frac{1}{3}$	One-third	0.33	33%
$\frac{50}{100}$	$\frac{1}{2}$	One-half	0.5 (0.50)	50%
$\frac{66}{100}$	$\frac{2}{3}$	Two-thirds	0.66	66%
$\frac{75}{100}$	$\frac{3}{4}$	Three-quarters	0.75	75%

RATIOS

A ratio is a way of describing a mixture of two or more components. For example, to mix substances A and B in the ratio 2:1 means that there are two parts of A to every one part of B, making three parts in total: $2 + 1 = 3$.

Ratio
A ratio is the relative sizes of two or more values.

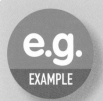

Let me show you an example...

A carton of 500 mL of concentrated juice has the instruction 'dilute 7 parts of water to 1 part of juice'. How much juice can be made from this bottle to give to a ward of patients during a heat wave? First we must pull out the information we need to work this out, and disregard the waffle.

Dilute 7 parts of water to 1 part of juice: this equates to 7:1, which means there are eight parts in total $(7 + 1 = 8)$.

Each part is worth 500 mL.

$$500 \times 1 = 500$$
$$500 \times 7 = 3500$$
$$3500 + 500 = 4000 \text{ mL in total.}$$

or

$$500 \text{ mL} \times 8 = 4000 \text{ mL (or 4 L)}$$

A strength of a solution may also be given as a ratio as 1 *in* 4. This means that 1 part of stock solution has been added in 3 parts of diluted solution.

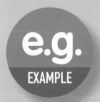

Let me show you an example...

EXAMPLE

The ratio 1 in 10 means that there is one part stock solution to every nine parts of dilutant: 10 parts in total. 10 minus 1 = 9 parts of dilutant, therefore 1 in 10 equates to 1:9.

Therefore 1 in 4 means 1 part of stock solution added in 4 parts of diluted solution.

1:3 means one part of stock solution added to three parts of dilutant.

Don't worry, let's look at another one: a learning disabilities nurse is taking her client to a swimming session. The pool is 20 m wide and 50 m long. What is the simplest ratio of the pool's width to its length?

Both the 20 and the 50 can be divided by 10:

$$20/10 = 2$$
$$50/10 = 5$$

Therefore, the simplest form of the ratio is **2:5**.

NOTE: adrenaline for anaphylaxis is expressed as 1:1000. This means that there is 1 mg for every 1 mL (1 mg/mL), which is equivalent to *1 g in every 1000 mL*. Therefore, if we were to administer 0.5 mg of the drug, we would need to give 0.5 mL.

Adrenaline for cardiac arrest is expressed as 1:10000. This means that there is 1 mg in 10 mL (or 0.1 mg for every 1 mL), or *1 g in 10000 mL*. As we administer the whole 10 mL of the drug, we are giving 10 times the volume than for anaphylaxis situations (10 mL).

See how you get on in Activity 1.5. Don't go peeking at the answers: have a go first!

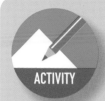

Activity 1.5

ACTIVITY

1   How much stock solution is present in 100 mL of diluted solution if expressing this as the ratio (i) 1 in 4 and (ii) 1:4?
2   How much stock solution is present in 5 L of diluted solution if expressing this as the ratio (i) 1 in 9 and (ii) 1:9?
3   How much stock solution is present in 550 mL of diluted solution if expressing this as the ratio (i) 1 in 10 and (ii) 1:10?
4   How much stock solution is present in 600 mL of diluted solution if expressing this as the ratio (i) 1 in 3 and (ii) 1:3?

AVERAGES

An average may be a mode, median, range or mean:

- **mode:** the most common figure in a series of figures;
- **median:** the figure in the centre of a series of values placed in order;
- **range:** the lowest to the highest value;
- **mean:** most commonly referred to as the 'average'. All values added together and divided by the number of units.

Let me show you an example...

e.g.

EXAMPLE

Brendan Topa's temperature during the day has been:

06:00	37.2°C (degrees Celsius)		
08:00	37.2°C	16:00	38.0°C
10:00	37.8°C	18:00	37.6°C
12:00	38.0°C	20:00	37.4°C
14:00	38.0°C	22:00	37.0°C

What is the mode?
38.0°C, as there are three recordings of this figure.

What is the median?

37.0	37.2	37.2	37.4	37.6
37.8	38.0	38.0	38.0	

The median is 37.6 when the values are placed in numerical order.

What is the range?
37.0–38.0: the smallest figure to the largest figure is the difference of one whole degree celsius (1°C).

What is the mean?

$$37.2 + 37.2 + 37.8 + 38.0 + 38.0 + 38.0 + 37.6 + 37.4 + 37.0 =$$
$$3382/9 \text{ (number of units)} = 37.57777 = 37.6°C$$

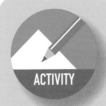

Activity 1.6

ACTIVITY

1   What is the mean average of Judith Goodman's intracranial pressure recordings? **NOTE:** intracranial pressure is the pressure of cerebrospinal fluid within the ventricles and subarachnoid space in the brain (I know, too much information!).

08:00	19 mmHg
09:00	19 mmHg
10:00	19.5 mmHg
11:00	18.0 mmHg
12:00	17 mmHg

KEY POINTS

- Revising calculations basics in decimals, metric measures, converting units, percentages, fractions, ratios and averages.
- Looking at how the strength of a solution can be expressed.

Chapter 2
. . . .
CALCULATIONS SELF-ASSESSMENT

Calculation Skills for Nurses, First Edition. Claire Boyd
© 2013 John Wiley & Sons, Ltd. Published 2013 by John Wiley & Sons Ltd.

LEARNING OUTCOMES

By the end of this chapter you will have a better understanding of your strengths and weaknesses relating to calculations and which sections of the book you should focus on to improve your abilities.

To assess your own calculations ability, it is recommended that you complete the self-assessment in this chapter. It will help you to identify any area that you have difficulty with, and that you need to brush up on. You can use a calculator but, first, why not have a go without one? Attempting the self-assessment will also help you to identify your own improvement when you attempt the Knowledge Tests at the end of this book, where everything we have learned throughout the book gets put into practice. Don't worry if you don't answer everything correctly first time around: just go back to Chapter 1 and rework the practice exercises, or, if you skipped that chapter, you may need to take a look at it now.

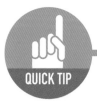

QUICK TIP

Remember the rule of 5s!

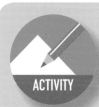

ACTIVITY

Activity 2.1

1   Round 0.78 to one decimal place.
2   Round 0.31 to one decimal place.
3   Round 4.72 to one decimal place.
4   Round 2.33 to one decimal place.
5   Round 9.45 to one decimal place.

6   Round 3.44 to one decimal place.
7   Round 2.418 to two decimal places.
8   Round 9.234 to two decimal places.
9   Round 0.915 to two decimal places.
10 Round 0.522 to two decimal places.
11 Round 2.340 to two decimal places.
12 Round 6.711 to two decimal places.
13 Round 0.8255 to three decimal places.
14 Round 1.5868 to three decimal places.
15 Change 39.4 to a whole number.
16 Change 31.7 to a whole number.
17 Change 39.9 to a whole number.

Remember: milligrams are *smaller* than grams.

18 Change 6000 mg into grams.
19 Change 0.7 micrograms into milligrams.
20 Change 9 micrograms into nanograms.

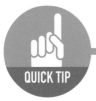

Remember: micrograms are *larger* than nanograms.

21 Change 0.03 g into milligrams.
22 Change 2.5 L into millilitres.

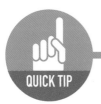

Remember: always make it clear if your answer has a decimal point.

23 Change 92 kg into grams.
24 Change 8 kg into grams.
25 Change 64.5 micrograms into milligrams.
26 Change 1527 micrograms into milligrams.
27 Change 0.02 mg into grams.
28 Change 1.2 mg into micrograms.
29 What is 25% of 500 mL?
30 What percentage is 92 of 150?
31 What is 10% of 233?
32 Change $\frac{4}{5}$ to a decimal with one decimal place.
33 Change $\frac{175}{5}$ to a decimal.
34 Change $\frac{1}{8}$ to a decimal with one decimal place.
35 How much stock solution is present in 200 mL of diluted solution if expressing this as a ratio of 1 in 5?
36 How much stock solution is present in 200 mL of diluted solution if expressing this as a ratio of 1:5?
37 How much stock solution is present in 600 mL of diluted solution if expressing this as a ratio of 1 in 3?

QUICK TIP

Remember: the mode is the most common figure in a set of figures.

38 What is the mode of 19, 19, 19.2, 20, 20.3 and 25?
39 What is the range of 6, 6.2, 9, 9.5 and 10?
40 What is the mean of 52, 52.4, 61, 67 and 70?

KEY POINT

- **Understanding your own strengths and weaknesses in calculations.**

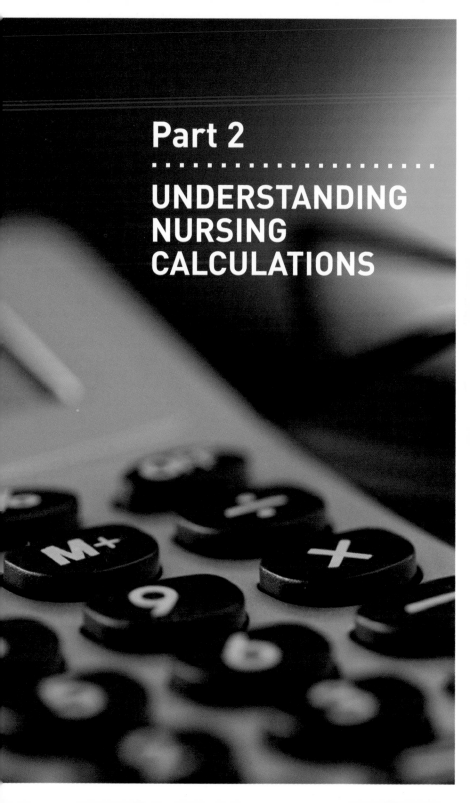

Part 2

. . . .

UNDERSTANDING NURSING CALCULATIONS

Chapter 3
. . . .
METRIC UNITS AND CONVERSIONS

Calculation Skills for Nurses, First Edition. Claire Boyd
© 2013 John Wiley & Sons, Ltd. Published 2013 by John Wiley & Sons Ltd.

LEARNING OUTCOMES

By the end of this chapter you should be familiar with the equivalences of weight and volume and converting from one unit to another.

We have already looked at the metric system and know the following:

Weight:	1 kilogram (kg)	= 1000 grams (g)
	1 gram (g)	= 1000 milligrams (mg)
	1 milligram (mg)	= 1000 micrograms
	1 microgram	= 1000 nanograms (ng)
	1 nanogram (ng)	= 1000 picograms (pg)
Volume:	1 litre (L)	= 1000 millilitres (mL)

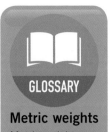

GLOSSARY

Metric weights
Metric weights are a decimal unit of weight based on the gram.

To convert LARGER units to smaller, the larger is multiplied.

To multiply by 1000 you move the decimal point three places to the right.

To convert smaller units to LARGER, the smaller is divided.

To divide by 1000 you move the decimal point three places to the left.

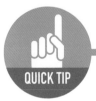

QUICK TIP

Remember the tip:

$\uparrow \div$ $\leftarrow \cdot$
$\downarrow \times$ $\cdot \rightarrow$

It may be necessary to convert imperial weights into metric weights, i.e. stones and pounds into kilograms, or vice versa. We need to know that:

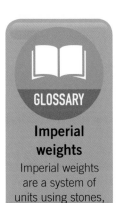

> 1 pound = 0.45 kg
> 1 stone = 6.35 kg, and
> 1 kg = 2.2 pounds (lb)

Imperial weights

Imperial weights are a system of units using stones, pounds and ounces.

For example, a patient weighs 9 stone, 5 lb. To convert this to the metric system, you could take the 9 stone and multiply this by 6.35 kg = 57.15 kg. Then take the 5 lb and multiply this by 0.45 kg = 2.25 kg. Add these together (57.15 + 2.25 kg). Therefore 9 stone, 5 lb = 59.40 kg.

Are you ready for some exercises? Who said no?

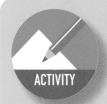

Activity 3.1

ACTIVITY

1   Change 3000 mg to grams.
2   Change 38 000 mL to litres.
3   Change 250 mL to litres.
4   Change 0.05 micrograms to milligrams.
5   Change 2000 g to kilograms.
6   Change 2500 mg to grams.
7   Change 0.3 mg to micrograms.
8   Change 6 micrograms to nanograms.
9   Change 1600 g to kilograms.
10 Change 0.375 mg to grams.
11 A patient weighs 15 stone, 10 lb. What is this in kilograms?
12 A patient weighs 82.55 kg and asks you what this is 'in old money', meaning in stones?

13 A patient has taken two doses of her 400 microgram glyceryl trinitrate spray. How many milligrams has she taken?

14 Change 0.075 mg to micrograms.

15 Change 935 grams to kilograms.

16 Digoxin tablets are presented as 125 micrograms. What is this in milligrams?

17 Change 1.4 litres to millilitres.

18 Change 27 mg to grams.

19 A patient has taken 0.75 g of medication. How much is this in milligrams?

20 Change 7 ng into picograms.

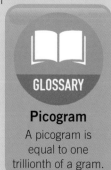

GLOSSARY

Picogram
A picogram is equal to one trillionth of a gram.

KEY POINTS

- Looking at metric and imperial weights.
- Looking at how to convert metric units and volumes.

Chapter 4
TABLETS AND CAPSULES

Calculation Skills for Nurses, First Edition. Claire Boyd
© 2013 John Wiley & Sons, Ltd. Published 2013 by John Wiley & Sons Ltd.

LEARNING OUTCOMES

By the end of this chapter you should be familiar with the formula 'what you want divided by what you have' (or similar wording) and calculating the total amount of tablets or capsules you require from a prescription.

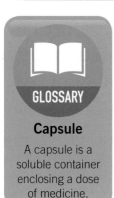

GLOSSARY

Capsule

A capsule is a soluble container enclosing a dose of medicine.

When working out how many tablets or capsules to administer for drug administration, some calculations can be quite simple:

Paracetamol is presented as 500 mg per tablet.

If a patient requires (is prescribed) 1000 mg we can see that two tablets are required (500 mg + 500 mg = 1000 mg). This is known as the calculations 'bundles' approach.

Or, we can use a formula:

$$\text{Number of tablets or capsules required} = \frac{\text{what you want}}{\text{what you've got}}$$

This means what you want divided by what you've got.

The formula approach comes into its own when we have more complicated calculations to work out. However, an understanding of the whys and wherefores of the problem must first be established: that is, what are we doing and why? We should always also be thinking around the box: does the answer look right? This means we should already have made a rough estimate (or 'guesstimation') of the answer.

NOTE: 'what you want' is what has been prescribed and we divide this by how the medication is presented in its blister pack or bottle, which is the 'what you've got' part.

It is important to use the wording that makes sense to you. Some people prefer to use these different expressions:

- What you need divided by what it comes in.
- Dose prescribed divided by dose you have available.

- Strength required divided by stock strength.
- What you desire divided by what is at hand.
- Amount desired divided by amount you have.

NOTE: it is important that when we are using a formula that all the metric units are the same. For example, if 'what you want' is in milligrams then the 'what you've got' has also got to be in milligrams. Now it should make sense why we have spent so much time on conversions in the previous chapters!

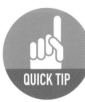

QUICK TIP

I think the wording I'll use is 'prescription divided by amount per tablet/capsule'. This makes sense to me.

Let me show you an example...

EXAMPLE

You pick up the prescription chart and see that a patient has been prescribed 225 mg of a drug. This is the **what you want** part of the formula.

Two tablets of the prescribed drug are in a blister pack in the stock cupboard. This is **what you've got** part of the formula. Each tablet is equal to 150 mg of the drug. Visualise yourself getting the drug out of the cupboard and popping the pills into a medicine pot. But you know two of these tablets will be too much, i.e. more than what the prescription asked for.

So you put the figures into the formula and, if using a calculator, input: 225 mg (what you want) divided by 150 mg (what you've got) = 1.5 = 1½ tablets. Therefore, one of the tablets needs to be split in half. Simples!

NOTE: remember what we said about cutting tablets in half: do so only if they are scored, and never cut a tablet into quarters.

Prescription chart

A prescription chart is a legal document under the UK Medicines Act 1968. It is a written direction of prescribed drugs.

Now have a go at working through some of these yourself, using the formula given above.

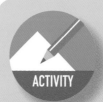

Activity 4.1a

In each case, calculate how many tablets or capsules are required.
1   Prescribed: 60 mg codeine phosphate; stock strength: 30 mg
2   Prescribed: 75 mg aspirin; stock strength: 150 mg aspirin
3   Prescribed: 225 mg ranitidine; stock strength: 150 mg
4   Prescribed: 0.5 micrograms daily (very small dose); stock strength: 250 mg (quite large dose). Is this really achievable? Remember, medics can make mistakes when writing prescriptions. Trust yourself.
5   What you want: 5 mg timolol maleate; what you've got: 10 mg
6   What you need: 15 mg nortriptyline; how it comes: 10 mg

Number of tablets: tablets may be available in different strengths and you should always give as few as possible, in the best combination (who likes swallowing pills at the best of times?).

Let me show you an example...

Tablets are presented as 10 mg, 5 mg, 2 mg and 1 mg. Working out the best combination for the following prescriptions show that:
1   Patient prescribed 11 mg = 10 mg + 1 mg = 2 tablets
2   Patient prescribed 8 mg = 5 mg + 2 mg + 1 mg = 3 tablets

3 Patient prescribed 12 mg = 10 mg + 2 mg = 2 tablets
4 Patient prescribed 4 mg = 2 mg + 2 mg = 2 tablets

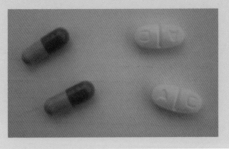

Want some more questions to practice on? Go on, you know you want to!

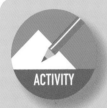

Activity 4.1b

ACTIVITY

1 Patient has been prescribed 125 micrograms of digoxin. You have 62.5 microgram tablets in stock. How many tablets do you give?

2 Warfarin tablets, in stock, are presented as 0.5 mg, 1 mg, 2 mg and 5 mg. Your patient is prescribed 9 mg. Which tablets do you administer for the required prescription?

3 Prescribed: 300 mg cimetidine. What you've got: 200 mg. How many tablets do you give?

4 Verapamil tablets come in strengths of 40 mg, 80 mg, 120 mg and 160 mg. A patient is prescribed 320 mg of the drug. Which tablets do you administer for the required prescription?

5 Prescribed: 75 mg thioridazine. You have 10 mg, 25 mg, 50 mg and 100 mg strengths in stock. Which tablets do you administer for the required prescription?

6 A patient has been prescribed 250 mg of chlorpropamide, to be administered with breakfast. Presently on the ward there are only 100 mg tablets obtainable. How many tablets do you give?

KEY POINTS

- Looking at the formula used to work out how many tablets or capsules to administer according to the prescribed prescription.
- Working out how to administer the smallest number of tablets or capsules for the dose prescribed.

Chapter 5

LIQUIDS AND INJECTABLES

Calculation Skills for Nurses, First Edition. Claire Boyd

LEARNING OUTCOMES

By the end of this chapter you should be familiar with the formula 'what you want divided by what you've got multiplied by the volume' (or similar wording) and be able to calculate the amount of drug (in millilitres) you require from a prescription. You will also have a working knowledge of how to use a calculator.

All injections (subcutaneous, intramuscular, intravenous, etc.) need to be in a liquid form (as it's difficult to push a dry tablet into someone's veins or muscle!).

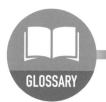

GLOSSARY

Intradermal injection
Liquid medication administered between the layers of the skin.

Subcutaneous injection
Liquid medication administered into the fatty tissue directly below the skin.

Intramuscular injection
Liquid medication inserted into the central area of a specific muscle.

Intravenous injection
Liquid medication administered through an access device directly into a vein.

So, these medications have been mixed in a transport medium (the liquid). Volume = liquid.

Let's imagine we have a 2 mg tablet. It is to be injected into the patient's muscle, so we use a mortar and pestle and crush the drug and then add the transport medium, water.

NOTE: we would not do this in practice! If we add 1 ml of water, the drug is said to be presented as 2 mg/1 mL. If we add 10 mL of water, then the drug is said to be 2 mg/10 mL. If we add 1000 mL (or 1 L) to the crushed tablet the drug is said to be 2 mg/1 L. The important thing to note that the drug amount has not changed, only the volume. Don't lose sight of the fact that in the last case we would still have a 2 mg tablet floating around in 1 L of liquid.

We can use the same formula as we used for dry dosages (see Chapter 4), but we now need to add the volume part to it:

$$\text{Volume of drug to be given} = \frac{\text{what you want}}{\text{what you've got}} \times \text{volume}$$

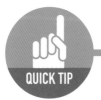

The answer will always be in millilitres now, as the drug is in a liquid form.

NOTE: this formula also works with other liquids, so it does not just apply to injectables; for example, cough syrups, elixirs and linctus.

As the drug is now in a liquid form, all our answers will now come in millilitres.

Let me show you an example...

e.g.
EXAMPLE

A patient has been prescribed 8 mg of morphine and stock ampoules contain 10 mg/mL. What I want = 8 mg, what I've got = 10 mg and what it comes in (volume) = 1 mL:

8 mg divided by 10 mg multiplied by 1 mL = 0.8 mL

So, I draw up 0.8 mL knowing that there is 8 mg of the drug in my syringe.

Looking at the whole picture, I know this looks about right as my answer should indeed be *under* the 1 mL mark, as this is how much liquid holds 10 mg of the drug, and I want less than this.

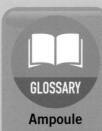

GLOSSARY

Ampoule
An ampoule is a sealed glass or plastic bulb containing a solution for hypodermic injection.

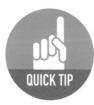

Liquid preparations are very common in baby and infant care.

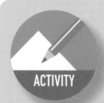

Activity 5.1

ACTIVITY

1 Gentamicin is dispensed as 80 mg in 2 mL. The prescription is to administer 50 mg of gentamicin. What volume of gentamicin do you administer?

2 Intravenous (or IV) metronidazole 500 mg is dispensed in a 100 ml bag. A 12-year-old child is prescribed 400 mg of metronidazole. What volume do you administer?

3 Heparin is dispensed as 25 000 units in 1 mL. 20 000 units of heparin is prescribed. What volume do you administer? (There is more about heparin, and units, in Chapter 6.)

4 Teicoplanin comes as 400 mg in 3 mL. A patient is prescribed 600 mg. How many millilitres do you give?

5 A patient is having an anaphylaxis episode (a severe allergic reaction) and requires adrenaline urgently. Adrenaline is presented as 1 mg in 1 mL (1:1000). You are required to administer 500 micrograms intramuscularly (or IM) now, and another 500 micrograms in 5 minutes' time. How much adrenaline (in milligrams and millilitres) do you administer in total?

6 Fluoxetine is presented as 20 mg/5 mL. A patient has been prescribed 30 mg. What volume do you administer?

7 Benzylpenicillin is presented in stock ampoules of 1.2 g in 6 mL of solution. A patient is prescribed 800 mg. What volume do you administer?

In the following, what volume of drug do you administer?

8 Prescribed: 250 mg oral suspension of amoxicillin; stock strength: 125 mg in 5 mL

9 Prescribed: atropine 0.5 mg; stock strength: 0.6 mg/mL

10 Prescribed: 1750 units of heparin; stock strength: 1000 units per mL

Some drugs have to be injected over a given time period, so as not to cause 'speed shock'. For example, furosemide should not exceed 4 mg of the drug over 1 minute.

GLOSSARY

Speed shock
Speed shock is a sudden, adverse physiological reaction to IV medication administered too quickly.

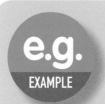

QUICK TIP

Speed shock can be caused by even very small amounts of a drug.

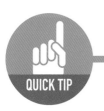

e.g.
EXAMPLE

Let me show you an example...

20 mg of furosemide is prescribed and drawn up, but the rate of administration should be no more than 4 mg of the drug over 1 minute, according to British National Formulary (BNF) instructions. This is the formula you may wish to use:

$$\text{Time needed to administer drug} = \frac{\text{dose prescribed}}{\text{rate}}$$

$$\frac{20 \text{ mg}}{4 \text{ mg}} = 5 \text{ min}$$

We will need to inject the furosemide over 5 minutes.

If using a calculator to make this calculation you take the amount prescribed and divide it by the rate: 20 mg divided by 4 mg = 5. The answer will be in minutes, as this is the formula for giving us times (in minutes).

CALCULATORS

If you wish to use a calculator, get used to inputting numbers into it and remember that some calculators are 'scientific', and so will have lots of buttons that you may not recognise. Some simple calculators do not have a square root button, but in case if you ever need to work out body surface areas it is a good idea to get a calculator with such a button. It looks like this:

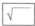

Whatever calculator you use, you will need to get used to using this tool, as many errors occur during the inputting stage. Always read the manufacturer's instructions after purchasing your calculator and practise using it with some sample questions to which you already know the answer before using it in real life. Remember, always ask yourself whether the answer looks right, and get it checked.

Let me show you an example...

To find 20% of 75, input:

| **2** | **0** | **×** | **7** | **5** | **%** | **=** | **15** |

Therefore 20% of 75 is 15. Did you notice that you did not need to press the equals (=) button (this may have lead to a wrong answer, and you would have got 1500).

To check our answer we can reverse our findings:

15	=	20%
15	=	20%
15	=	20%
15	=	20%
15	=	20%
		100%

Five bundles of 15 make our 75, which makes up our 100%, so 15 is correct.

NOTE: if your calculator does not have a percentage button, then you just input: $20/100 \times 75 = 15$.

KEY POINTS

- Looking at the formula used to work out the amount of millilitres to administer volumes according to the prescribed prescription.
- Becoming conversant with the different types of injection.
- Understanding the basic principles of speed shock in relation to administering IV medications.
- How to input data into a calculator.

Chapter 6
....
SYRINGES AND MENISCUS

Calculation Skills for Nurses, First Edition. Claire Boyd
© 2013 John Wiley & Sons, Ltd. Published 2013 by John Wiley & Sons Ltd.

LEARNING OUTCOMES

By the end of this chapter you will be aware of the calibrations attributed to the various-sized syringes and syringe types. You will also have an understanding of injection needles and the meniscus effect.

GLOSSARY

Enteral route

The enteral route refers to the administration of a drug directly into the stomach and intestines.

Analgesia

Analgesia is medication that reduces or eliminates pain.

Syringes are used to inject medications via the intradermal (within the skin), subcutaneous, intramuscular or intravenous routes. In the neurosciences medics also use a route known as intrathecal, or within the meninges of the spinal cord. There are many reasons why we would need to give patients their medication with a syringe and needle using one of these routes. For example, patients may be unable to swallow and or unable to tolerate medications and fluid via the oral enteral route, or the prescribed medication may not come in an oral formulation (such as insulin), being destroyed by chemicals in the intestine. An injection of analgesia is more quickly absorbed by the body than a tablet or capsule, which is again the rationale for an injectable format to be chosen. Not all syringes will need to have a needle attached when administering a drug, as we do have oral syringes, often used in paediatrics to measure and administer oral medications. *Oral syringes are not the same as other syringes.*

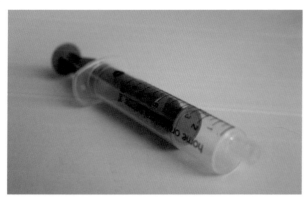

An oral syringe.

THE SYRINGE

The syringe consists of a barrel to contain the liquid that is drawn up, with calibrations marked along the outer surface.

The moveable plunger is contained inside the barrel and has an end tip. Pulling this plunger back sucks fluid into the barrel and pushing this in, or forward, expels this fluid.

The syringe has an end tip, or different varieties and placement, in order for a needle to be attached.

Types of Syringe

Luer-lock   This is used for secure connections, whereby the needle is screwed onto the syringe.

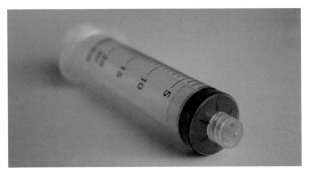

A Luer-lock syringe.

Eccentric Luer-slip   This is where the nozzle is off-centre to allow closer application to the skin.

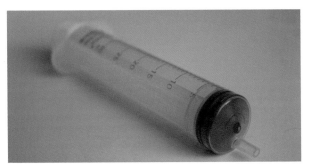

An eccentric Luer-slip syringe.

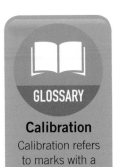

GLOSSARY

Calibration

Calibration refers to marks with a standard scale of readings.

Concentric Luer-slip   This is used for all other applications. The nozzle is in the centre.

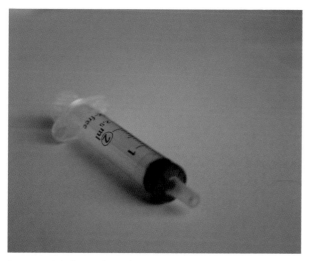

A concentric Luer-slip syringe.

Syringes come in various sizes with different calibrations:

> 1 mL syringes have divisions of 0.01 mL
>
> 2 mL syringes have divisions of 0.1 mL
>
> 5 mL syringes have divisions of 0.2 mL
>
> 10 mL, 20 mL and 50 mL syringes have 1 mL divisions

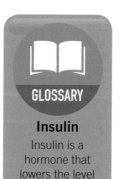

GLOSSARY

Insulin

Insulin is a hormone that lowers the level of glucose in the blood.

Insulin

Insulin syringes are used to administer insulin, which is prepared as units per millilitre, in vials that contain 100 units/mL: these are known as multi-dose vials. The standard insulin syringe is calibrated in 2-unit divisions up to 100 units. Patients may require only a small dose (less than 50 units) and so there are also low-dose syringes available which are graduated in 1-unit divisions up to 50 units (in 0.5 mL syringes).

Heparin

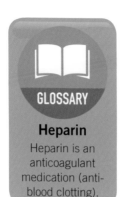

Like insulin, heparin is prescribed in units and drawn up in 1 mL syringes, or comes in pre-filled syringes. Heparin is available in single or multi-dose vials, in variable strengths, such as:

1000 units/mL

5000 units/mL

25 000 units/mL

5000 units/5 mL

25 000 units/5 mL

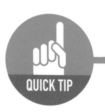

QUICK TIP

You may still see some medics writing units on prescription charts as IU, meaning International Units. This can be confused with IV for intravenous, so the word units is now preferred.

Don't confuse units with millilitres!

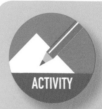

ACTIVITY

Activity 6.1

1   Mark 30.5 mL on this 50 mL syringe.

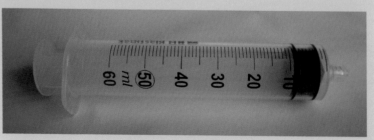

2   Mark 0.75 mL on this syringe.

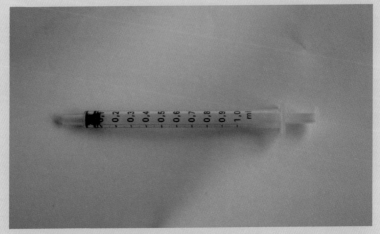

3   How much has been drawn up in this syringe?

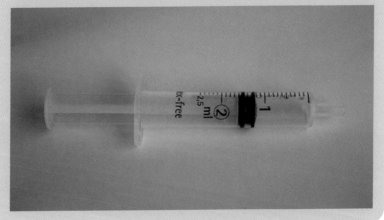

NOTE: a syringe should ideally only be filled to 75% capacity. This is in order for any re-adjustments to be made when drawing up, and is especially true when injecting into muscle, and drawing back to establish that we are not about to inject the medication into a blood vessel. You may have noticed that the 50 mL syringe goes up to 60 mL graduations.

When drawing up medication from an ampoule or vial, ideally a specialised blunt filter needle should be used, but these may not be readily available. Therefore it is considered best practice to use a quite small needle, to reduce the effect of drawing up shards of glass or particles of the rubber from these receptacles. After the medication has been drawn up the blue needle should be replaced with the appropriate-sized needle prior to administration.

Needles Come in Gauge Sizes

QUICK TIP

The larger the number on a needle, the smaller the needle.

The three most common needles you may use in practice are:

40 mm (21 gauge, or g) = quite large needle

25 mm (23 g) = quite small needle

16 mm (25 g) = very small needle, often used for subcutaneous injections

The higher the gauge, the finer the bore.

INJECTIONS

The routes most commonly used for the administration of injections are the subcutaneous (SC; beneath the skin), the intramuscular (IM; into muscle) and the intravenous (IV; into a vein) routes. The buttocks tend to be the most common site for IM injections, but due to the presence of nerves in this region, especially the sciatic nerve, this may give rise to nerve damage. The sites used for IM injections tend to be the deltoid (arm), ventrogluteal, dorsogluteal (both buttock muscles, the upper outer quadrant of the buttock) and vastus lateralis (middle outer aspect of the thigh) muscles. Study these muscles in a book on anatomy and physiology.

Subcutaneous injections are administered into the subcutaneous tissue rather than a muscle. Medications administered into this tissue have a slow and steady absorption and blood vessels and nerves are minimal in these areas. The sites most commonly used for subcutaneous injections are the middle outer aspect of the upper arm, the middle anterior aspect of the thigh or the anterior abdominal wall just below the umbilicus.

Needles for Injection

Needles consist of a hub and the tip of the needle is bevelled: this is a 'cut out'. The bevel is uppermost when injecting for intradermal injections, and downwards for all other injections. IM injections into the buttocks tend to be with either a 21 g or 23 g needle. The size of needle depends on the patient's size: 21 g is suitable for most adults and obese adults, whereas 23 g is suitable for very thin adults.

For IM injections into the thigh and arm the 23 g is suitable for most adults.

For SC injections the 25 g tends to be used.

Meniscus

Surface tension of a liquid causes it to produce a curved surface as the liquid climbs up the sides of a container. This is called the meniscus. To accurately measure the liquid in a medicine pot or syringe you read the bottom of the curve of the meniscus, where it is at its lowest, in the middle (the bottom of the meniscus), not the top of the curve (top of the meniscus).

Activity 6.2

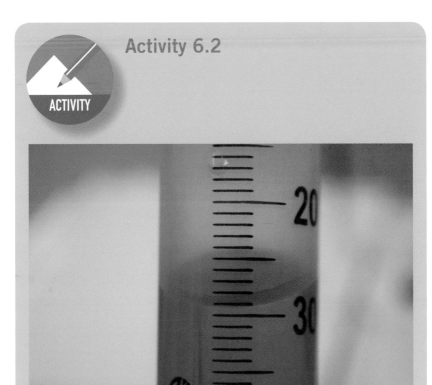

What is the reading on this syringe?

Practice reading the meniscus levels of medications in syringes and medicine pots: always read the lowest level of the curve, and always hold the container at eye level to obtain an accurate reading.

KEY POINTS

- Looking at syringes, including the oral syringe.
- Looking at injection needle gauge sizes and choosing the correct gauge size for injections.
- Understanding the meniscus effect.

Chapter 7
DISPLACEMENT VALUES

Calculation Skills for Nurses, First Edition. Claire Boyd
© 2013 John Wiley & Sons, Ltd. Published 2013 by John Wiley & Sons Ltd.

LEARNING OUTCOMES

By the end of this chapter you will have an understanding of the displacement value when reconstituting drugs.

GLOSSARY

Paediatric care
Relating to the care of infants, children and adolescents.

Neonatal care
Relating to the care of newborn babies.

Some drugs, such as those needing to be freeze-dried to a powder for storage, require reconstitution with liquid prior to being administered. When dissolved in the liquid, the powder will take up space and will have to be added to the final volume when drawn up into a syringe; this additional volume must be taken into account when thinking about how much liquid to draw into the syringe. Displacement values come into play when less than a whole ampoule or vial needs to be reconstituted. This is a frequent occurrence in paediatric and neonatal care.

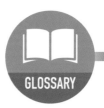

GLOSSARY

Reconstituting drugs
Reconstitution refers to building up again; to reconstruct, to restore something to its original state by adding water.

Amoxicillin
Amoxicillin is an antibiotic of the penicillin type.

Let me show you an example...

To give a dose of 125 mg amoxycillin from a 250 mg vial:
- the displacement value for amoxycillin 250 mg is 0.2 mL;
- if you add 4.8 mL of fluid, you will then have a total of 5 mL in the vial (4.8 mL + 0.2 mL displacement value), giving you 250 mg in 5 mL;
- therefore, to administer 125 mg, you will need to administer 2.5 mL of the solution.

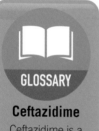

GLOSSARY

Ceftazidime

Ceftazidime is a cephalosporin antibiotic used to treat enterobacterial infections.

Let's Explain this Another Way

A patient is prescribed 1.5 g ceftazidime BD (which means twice a day), administered as a bolus. You have been provided with a 2 g vial, which needs to be reconstituted (with water for injection, or WFI) to make a total volume of 10 mL. The displacement value is 1.5 mL/2 g vial.

To make up to a total of 10 mL, you need to add 8.5 mL WFI. This is because the displacement value takes up 1.5 mL (10 mL − 1.5 mL = 8.5 mL).

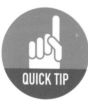

QUICK TIP

This can be expressed as 'volume to be added equals dilutant volume minus displacement value'.

Now that you have a volume of 10 mL, how many millilitres of this solution will you draw up to administer 1.5 g of the drug?

If you were to draw all the liquid from the ampoule, you would have 10 mL in the syringe. However, you do not want this full amount because the vial contained 2 g, and the prescribed dose is 1.5 g. So, use my formula to find out how much of this liquid you would need to draw out to make the prescribed dose of 1.5 g.

$$\text{Volume of drug to be given} = \frac{\text{what you want}}{\text{what you've got}} \times \text{volume}$$

$$\frac{1.5 \text{ g}}{2 \text{ g}} \times 10 \text{ mL} = 7.5 \text{ mL}$$

So 7.5 mL contains the required amount ordered on the prescription: 1.5 g.

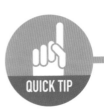

QUICK TIP

This means that if I had been asked to reconstitute a drug in 4 mL WFI, this is the *total* that will be in the syringe at the end, ready for administration, so that's why I don't actually add 4 mL of WFI to the vial.

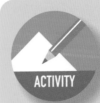

QUICK TIP

For explanations of Latin abbreviations like BD, and others, see the list at the start of the book.

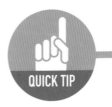

ACTIVITY

Activity 7.1

1 A patient is prescribed 600 mg of benzylpenicillin. The drug is presented in 600 mg vials, which need to be reconstituted (medic's instructions) in 4 mL of water for injection. Displacement value is 0.4 mL/600 mg. How much water do you add to the vial?

2   A small child has been prescribed 350 mg ceftriaxone IV daily. The drug
    is presented in 1 g vials and requires reconstituting in water for injection
    (WFI) to make a total volume of 10 mL. Displacement value is 0.8 mL/g.
    What volume of WFI needs to be added to the vial to make a total of
    10 mL?

3   A 1 gram vial of cefotaxime IV needs to be reconstituted to 4 mL water for
    injection (WFI). The displacement value is 0.5 mL/g. What volume of WFI
    do you add to the vial?

4   A vial of flucloxacillin 250 mg needs to be reconstituted in 5 mL WFI.
    Displacement value = 0.2 mL to every 250 mg vial. What volume of WFI do
    you add to this vial?

KEY POINTS

- Looking at reconstituting freeze-dried drugs from a
  powder to a liquid.
- Understanding the importance of displacement when
  reconstituting drugs.

Chapter 8

· ·

DOSAGES ACCORDING TO BODY WEIGHT

Calculation Skills for Nurses, First Edition. Claire Boyd
© 2013 John Wiley & Sons, Ltd. Published 2013 by John Wiley & Sons Ltd.

LEARNING OUTCOMES

By the end of this chapter you will be familiar with how to titrate drug dosages according to body weight using 'weight (kg) multiplied by dose' formula.

GLOSSARY

Titration

The process of determining the concentration of a substance in solution to be administered to individuals according to body weight.

Some drugs need to be titrated according to a person's body weight. For example, a small child will require a much smaller dose of a drug than a large adult. The formula we can use to titrate the amount is weight (in kg) multiplied by dose:

Correct dosage = weight (kg) × dose

For example, if we had a small lady weighing 55 kg and a 2 mg drug, we could use the above formula, which works out as 55 kg × 2 mg = 110 mg of the drug, either per day or per hour, according to the prescription. A 70 kg patient would require 140 mg of the drug either per day or per hour (that's 70 × 2).

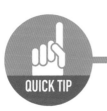

QUICK TIP

This formula is used a lot in paediatric patients, neonates, critical care and the elderly.
It is always important to get your answer checked.

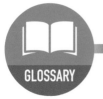

GLOSSARY

Critical care

Critical care relates to the specialised care of patients whose conditions are life-threatening and who require comprehensive care and monitoring.

Activity 8.1

1   A patient weighing 70 kg is prescribed 10 mg/kg/h of a drug. How many milligrams per hour of the drug does the patient need? Note that h means hour.
2   Paracetamol is prescribed as 10 mg/kg daily and can be given every 8 hours. How much would you give to a baby weighing 2.5 kg, both daily and every 8 hours?
3   Ranitidine is prescribed as 2 mg/kg. How many milligrams will be prescribed to a baby weighing 0.57 kg?

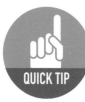

If baby's weight is in grams, you will need to convert to kilograms to fit the formula.

4   A drug is prescribed as 30 mg/kg. The patient weighs 48 kg. What dose should be given? If this dose is to be administered in three equal doses daily, how much is given in each dose?

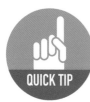

Drugs may be administered:

> **OD** = once a day
> **BD** = twice a day
> **TDS** = three times a day
> **QDS** = four times a day

Some drugs may need to be administered more frequently than this (e.g. hourly), or less frequently than this (e.g. once every 3 months).

If you have worked out a daily dose amount, this may need to be divided into two, three or four even doses depending on the prescription instructions.

The meanings of these Latin abbreviations, and more, are also given at the start of the book.

5 A 15 kg child is prescribed a drug 40 mg/kg/day, four doses daily. Calculate a single dose.

6 A 20 kg child is prescribed a drug 80 mg/kg/day, four doses daily. Calculate a single dose.

7 Flucloxacillin is prescribed as 100 mg/kg/day, four doses daily. The patient weighs 58 kg. Calculate a single dose.

8 A patient weighs 92 kg. A drug is prescribed as 60 mg/kg/day, four doses per day. Calculate a single dose.

9 A patient weighs 35 kg. Capreomycin sulphate is prescribed as 20 mg/kg/day, three doses per day. Calculate a single dose.

10 A 20 kg child is prescribed 45 mg/kg/day of a drug, four doses per day. Calculate a single dose.

KEY POINTS

- Looking at calculating dosages according to body weight using the formula 'weight (kg) multiplied by dose'.
- Understanding the importance of drug titration.
- Looking at Latin abbreviations for administering drugs.

Chapter 9

....

DRIP RATES

Calculation Skills for Nurses, First Edition. Claire Boyd
© 2013 John Wiley & Sons, Ltd. Published 2013 by John Wiley & Sons Ltd.

LEARNING OUTCOMES

By the end of this chapter you should be familiar with working out drip-rate calculations using the formula 'volume divided by time multiplied by drops per millilitres divided by minutes per hour'.

Some patients require IV hydration in the form of a 'drip', which is administered through a line, known as an administration set. Best practice is always to put these fluids through a pump, but sometimes they can be delivered via gravity, meaning without a pump.

This calculation is required for gravity-fed infusions (the manual method for working out the infusion rate), and gives us an answer in drops per minute. In order to calculate the rate in drops per minute the following formula is used:

$$\text{Rate} = \frac{\text{volume}}{\text{time in hours}}$$

$$\times \frac{\text{drops per millilitre}}{\text{minutes per hour}}$$

Let's break the formula up into parts to make sense of it: The **volume** is the amount that has been prescribed; for example, 1 L of sodium chloride 0.9%. The **time in hours** is also what has been prescribed by the medic, and may be something like 'to be given over 8 hours'.

Minutes per hour is always 60, as there are only 60 minutes in an hour! The **drops per millilitre** depends on the type of fluid being infused and the type of giving set (or administration set) in use. In general check the infusion set packaging for the flow rate of the set.

Blood administration or standard giving set:

- Blood and 'thick' fluids   15 drops/mL
- Clear fluids   20 drops/mL

Microdrip or paediatric giving set, sometimes referred to as a microdrop burette:

- Clear fluids   60 drops/mL

GLOSSARY

Burette

A burette is a glass or plastic tube with fine graduations and a stopcock at the bottom.

Putting this all together, we work this out as:

Volume amount divided by time in hours multiplied by drops per millilitre (depends on the infusate) divided by minutes per hour (always 60)

When we ave worked out our answer we need to count the 'drip rate', adjusting this accordingly until we get the correct number of drops dripping into the drip-rate chamber.

Let me show you an example...

EXAMPLE

A patient is to receive 1 L of 5% glucose in 8 hours. Calculate the rate in drops per minute, using a standard giving set (20 drops/mL).

Using the above formula:

$$\text{Rate} = \frac{1000 \text{ mL}}{8 \text{ hours}} \times \frac{20 \text{ drops/mL}}{60 \text{ minutes}} = \frac{1000}{8} \times \frac{20}{60}$$

$$= 41.6$$

$$= 42 \text{ drops per minute (to the nearest drop)}$$

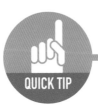

You need to use the rule of 5s to get a whole drop as your answer.

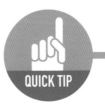

Work this out all in one go on your calculator: 1000 divided by 8 multiplied by 20 divided by 60 = 41.666666.

The answer to this question is 41.6, but as we can't count part of a drop, we follow the rule of 5s, and round 41.6 up to the next whole number: in this case 42 drops per minute. When we set up the equipment, we count 42 drops, dripping into the drip chamber: speeding it up, or slowing the drips down using the roller clamp. The end of the administration set gets attached to a cannula on the patient, so that the medication gets delivered intravenously.

Activity 9.1

1   1.5 L of sodium chloride has been prescribed to run over 12 hours. Using a standard IV administration set delivering 20 drops/mL, how many drops per minute will the infusion run at?

2   Calculate the following to the nearest whole drop: 420 mL of blood is to be given to a patient over 4 hours using a blood administration set (15 drops/mL).

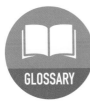

GLOSSARY

Hartmann's solution

This is a solution containing sodium chloride, sodium lactate and phosphates of calcium and potassium, used intravenously.

3 150 mL of Hartmann's solution is prescribed to run over 6 hours. The microdrip administration set delivers 60 drops/mL. How many drops per minute will the infusion be set to run?

4 A patient has been prescribed 350 mL of blood to be administered over 3 hours. Calculate the rate in drops per minute.

5 A patient is to receive half a litre of dextrose 5% over 6 hours. Calculate the rate in drops per minute.

6 A patient has two intravenous lines inserted. One line is running at 25 mL/hour and the other at 30 mL/hour. What volume of fluid does the patient receive in a 24 period?

7 A patient is prescribed 1 L of sodium chloride 0.9% to run over 6 hours. Calculate the drip rate in drops per minute.

8 1.5 L of clear fluid is prescribed to run over 10 hours. Calculate the drip rate in drops per minute.

9 A unit of packed red cells of blood (260 mL) is to be administered over 2 hours. Calculate the drip rate in drops per minute.

10 A unit of 250 mL of packed red blood cells is being administered. Half of this unit has already been transfused. A doctor has requested that the remaining half unit be administered over 1 hour. Calculate the drip rate in drops per minute.

11 A small baby has been prescribed 200 mL of 5% glucose to run over 2 hours through a microdrop administration set. Calculate the drip rate in drops per minute.

12 150 mL of 0.9% saline has been prescribed to run over 4 hours through a microdrop administration set. Calculate the drip rate in drops per minute.

NOTE: when administering blood, or potassium additives to a bag of fluid, a volumetric pump must always be used. This is a specialised piece of machinery with an alarm to alert staff when the fluids have 'gone through' or if air has got into the tubing, etc.

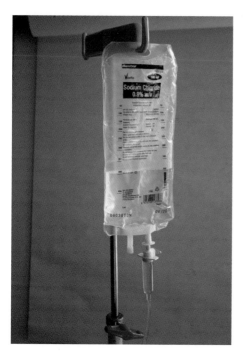

Bags of fluids (such as sodium chloride 0.9%) are best administered via a volumetric pump. This also applies to quantities of fluid over 50 mL. A volumetric pump delivers fluid in whole millilitres per hour, after you have programmed it with the information of how much liquid is to go through and at what time.

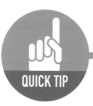

QUICK TIP

Having a formula makes working out drip rates easy!

KEY POINTS

- How to use a formula to work out drip rates on gravity infusions.
- Looking at blood administration sets.
- Looking at standard administration sets.
- Looking at microdrip and burette IV fluid devices.

Chapter 10

DRIP-RATE DURATION

Calculation Skills for Nurses, First Edition. Claire Boyd
© 2013 John Wiley & Sons, Ltd. Published 2013 by John Wiley & Sons Ltd.

LEARNING OUTCOMES

By the end of this chapter you should be familiar with the formula for working out drip-rate durations: 'volume divided by rate multiplied by drops per millilitre divided by 60 minutes'.

It is sometimes necessary to work out how long an infusion will take to complete, or 'go through', before the bag is empty. The formula we use for this is very similar to the drip-rate formula, but as we already know how many drops per minute are going through, so this gets added to the formula as 'rate of infusion' or 'drops per minute':

$$\text{Drip-rate duration} = \frac{\text{volume}}{\substack{\text{rate of infusion} \\ \text{(drops per minute)}}} \times \frac{\text{drops per millilitre}}{60 \text{ minutes}}$$

QUICK TIP

You need to know how to work out these rates manually in case a pump is not available.

It may also be necessary to adjust the rate, using the roller clamp, to speed up or slow down the infusion.

Remember: this formula is for manual application of fluids, as pumps deliver fluids in millilitres per hour.

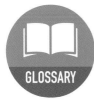

Roller clamp
A roller clamp is part of the IV administration line that adjusts the drip rate (speeds up or slows down the flow rate).

GLOSSARY

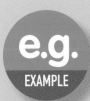

Let me show you an example...

e.g.
EXAMPLE

A patient has received approximately 800 mL of his sodium chloride 0.9% w/v prescription from a 1 L bag of fluid in 6 hours. As this is clear fluids, the administration set delivers 20 drops per millilitre. The fluid was dripping at 42 drops per minute. 'How long has the infusion got left to go?' someone asks. This is how I work out the answer:

First I look at the bag and estimate that there is 200 mL left to infuse. Then I put the information into my formula:

$$\frac{200}{42} \times \frac{20}{60} = 1.587$$

Which means that there is just over 1½ hours left to infuse these fluids.

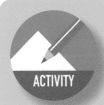

Activity 10.1

ACTIVITY

1 A patient is to have 3 L of clear fluid in 24 hours. He has received 1500 mL in 8 hours. How many drops per minute are required to correct the infusion?

2 600 mL of fluid is dripping at 20 drops per minute. The IV set delivers 15 drops per millilitre. How long will the infusion take?

3 1000 mL of fluid is dripping at 20 drops per minute. The IV set delivers 15 drops per millilitre. How long will the infusion take?

4 A patient is to have 2 L of clear fluid in 24 hours. She has received 1500 mL in 6 hours. How many drops per minute are required to correct the infusion?

5 Volume of clear fluid = 1000 mL. Rate of infusion = 43 drops per minute. How long will the infusion take?

KEY POINT

• How to use a formula to work out drip-rate durations.

Chapter 11

· · · · · · · · · · · · · · · · · · ·

SYRINGE DRIVERS
AND PUMPS

Calculation Skills for Nurses, First Edition. Claire Boyd
© 2013 John Wiley & Sons, Ltd. Published 2013 by John Wiley & Sons Ltd.

LEARNING OUTCOMES

By the end of this chapter you should be familiar with working out calculations in millilitres per hour using the formula 'volume divided by time' and in measuring millimetres per hour.

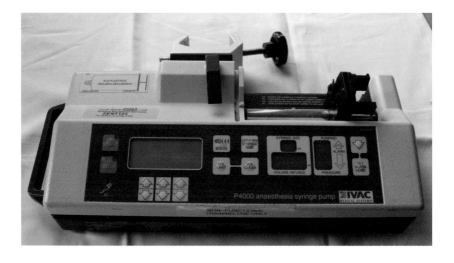

Some drugs, such as heparin and analgesics, need to be administered via specialised machinery, such as a syringe pump. These devices deliver set amounts of very concentrated drugs and with low flow rates, usually anything from 0.1 to 99 mL/hour. It is important that anyone using these devices undergoes specialist training, as many different devices are used in clinical areas.

The formula for working out the intravenous infusion rate in millilitres per hour for syringe pumps is:

$$\text{Infusion rate (mL/hour, pump)} = \frac{\text{amount of fluid (mL)}}{\text{infusion time (hours)}}$$

This can be shortened to $\dfrac{\text{volume}}{\text{time}}$.

So, if I had 48 mL of fluid in my syringe to be delivered over 24 hours, I would input:

$$\frac{48\ \text{mL}}{24\ \text{hours}} = 2\ \text{mL/hour}$$

Therefore I would set the machine to deliver 2 mL per hour, and after 24 hours my syringe would be empty.

Now, let's see how you get with the following questions.

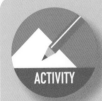

Activity 11.1

ACTIVITY

1   Mr Smith is prescribed a **total volume** of 48 mL of heparin and dilutant to be administered over 24 hours. What is the infusion rate in millilitres per hour? If you get this one wrong, you will know that you have missed the explanations (see above!).

2   An insulin infusion containing 50 units of human Actrapid has been diluted with 50 mL of sodium chloride, which has been running at:

   3 mL/hour for 2 hours
   3.5 mL/hour for 3 hours
   2 mL/hour for 1 hour
   2.5 mL/hour for 1 hour
   4 mL/hour for 2 hours

   How many units of Actrapid insulin in total has the patient received?

3   1 L of normal saline is to be administered over 8 hours. How many millilitres per hour is this?

4   A patient is to receive half a litre of normal saline over 6 hours. How many millilitres an hour should the pump be set?

5   Heparin has been diluted with an infusate to make a total volume of 48 mL in the syringe. This is to be given over 12 hours. At what rate should the infusion pump be set?

6   Over a 12 hour period, a patient is to receive 1 L of dextrose. At what rate should the infusion pump be set?

7   A patient is to receive 24 mL of medication over 12 hours. At what rate should the infusion pump be set?

8   100 mL of metronidazole has been prescribed to run over half an hour. At what rate should the infusion pump be set?

9   80 mL of fluid is to be infused over 30 minutes. At what rate should the infusion pump be set?

10 75 mL of fluid needs to be infused over 20 minutes. Calculate the rate in millilitres per hour.

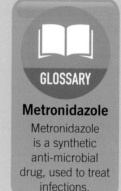

GLOSSARY

Metronidazole

Metronidazole is a synthetic anti-microbial drug, used to treat infections.

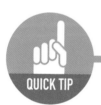

QUICK TIP

Watch out! She's trying to catch us out: did you notice that question 10 is presented in minutes and the answer needs to be in millilitres per *hour*. Don't forget to multiply the 75 mL by 60 minutes to get the hourly rate.

$$\frac{\text{Volume (mL)} \times 60 \text{ minutes}}{\text{Time (minutes)}}$$

This method can be used when infusion times are given in minutes, and when medication has been added to a burette. Do you remember from Chapter 9 that a burette is a microdrip administration set, administered via a volumetric pump? We use this when we need to convert our answer to millilitres per hour.

Let me show you an example...

Penicillin has been added to a burette to make up a total volume of 40 mL. The infusion time is 20 minutes.

$$\frac{40\ mL \times 60\ minutes}{20\ minutes} = 120\ mL/hour$$

Activity 11.2

Medications have been added to each of these burettes to make a total volume of fluid. Calculate the required pump settings in millilitres per hour.

1. Penicillin added to make a total volume of 50 mL of fluid. To be administered over 20 minutes.
2. Penicillin added to make a total volume of 100 mL of fluid. To be administered over 30 minutes.
3. Flucloxacillin added to make a total volume of 100 mL of fluid. To be administered over half an hour.
4. Vancomycin added to make a total volume of 120 mL of fluid. To be administered over 50 minutes.
5. Gentamicin added to make a total volume of 80 mL of fluid. To be administered over 50 minutes.
6. Ranitidine added to make a total volume of 60 mL of fluid. To be administered over 45 minutes.

Did you notice that the dosage of medication did not have a bearing on our calculations? The drug amount was incorporated into the total volume amount for you, and it is this that we put into the formula. For instance, in question 1 the penicillin dose was 600 mg, which equated to 5 mL, but you did not have this information, and did not need it to work out the answer in this case. We therefore added this to 45 mL of fluid in the burette to make a total volume of 50 mL.

SYRINGE DRIVERS

These pumps are usually small and compact, can be battery-operated and may be carried by the patient. Some devices deliver continuous subcutaneous infusions, at either an hourly rate (millilitres per hour) or a daily rate (over 24 hours).

Here's an example of an hourly rate prescription:

A patient is prescribed a dose of diamorphine at 2.5 mg/hour. Work out the dose for 24 hours.
2.5 mg/hour for 24 hours = 2.5 mg × 24 hours = 60 mg/ 24 hours

Here's an example of an hourly rate in millilitres per hour:

The prescription may state that the patient is to receive 60 mg of diamorphine in 24 hours, so no calculation is needed as this is a straightforward dose.

Millimetres Per Hour

Syringe drivers do not rely on the amount of liquid, or volume, in the syringe, but on the length of the column of fluid. The front of the syringe driver should have a millimetre scale, which is used to measure the length of fluid from the upper edge of the plunger to the 'zero' mark at the top of the syringe. So, the size of the syringe is vitally important to the calculation.

If the syringe contains 8 mL of fluid then the measurement will be 48 mm.

Here's an example of setting the rate in millimetres per hour.

If the prescription is to be delivered over 24 hours, you use the 48 mm (amount of fluid length in the syringe = 8 mL) and divide this by the infusion time in days:

$$\frac{48 \text{ mm}}{24 \text{ hours}} = 2 \text{ mm/hour}$$

Even though 48 mm is not the volume, for these syringe drivers some individuals use the formula:

$$\frac{\text{Volume}}{\text{Time}}$$

This could be said to be the same as:

$$\frac{\text{Length 48 mm}}{\text{Time}}$$

These calculations are very advanced and will always require double-checking and two individuals to work them out. If you are a student, get involved as a third checker to gain experience. It is always easier to be shown how to make these advanced calculations in the workplace, but let's see how you get on with following my steps.

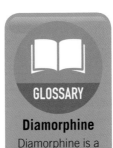

GLOSSARY

Diamorphine

Diamorphine is a powerful heroin opiod drug.

Cyclizine

Cyclizine is an anti-emetic drug often prescribed to treat nausea and/ or vomiting.

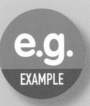

EXAMPLE

Let me show you an example...

A prescription for diamorphine 20 mg and cyclizine 50 mg is to be given over 24 hours. The syringe driver, which holds a 10 mL syringe, is set to deliver 2 mm/hour. The length of 8 mL in the syringe is measured up as 48 mm. Diamorphine is available in powder form in 10 mg ampoules. Cyclizine is available in ampoules containing 50 mg/2 mL. How is the solution made up?

STEP 1: calculate the total solution required to be delivered at 2 mm/hour.

2 mm/hour × 24 hour = 48 mm

48 mm = 8 mL total solution

STEP 2: calculate the volume of water for injection required to dilute the diamorphine.

Cyclizine 50 mg = 2 mL

8 mL – 2 mL = 6 mL for the diamorphine

Dilute the 20 mg of diamorphine with 6 mL of water. Therefore the syringe contains 8 mL. 6 mL of this is diamorphine and 2 mL of this is cyclizine, making up the total volume of 8 mL. This equates to 48 mm.

Don't worry if you found this too difficult, as you can always come back to look at syringe drivers at a later date. But if you do feel like a challenge, have a go at the next question.

Activity 11.3

ACTIVITY

1   The prescription is diamorphine 30 mg and cyclizine 50 mg/1 mL, which is to be administered over 24 hours in a syringe driver holding a 10 mL syringe.
   (a)   How much water for injection would be required to make up an 8 mL syringe containing cyclizine alone?
   (b)   If every 10 mg of diamorphine is to be diluted with 1 mL of water for injection, how much water is required to make the 8 mL syringe of diamorphine and cyclizine together?
   (c)   What rate should the syringe driver be set to deliver the 8 mL over 24 hours?

KEY POINTS

- Looking at syringe drivers and pumps.
- How to work out intravenous rates in millilitres per hour.
- How to work out rates according to devices delivering drugs in mm/hour.

Chapter 12
. . . .
PAEDIATRIC NURSING

Calculation Skills for Nurses, First Edition. Claire Boyd
© 2013 John Wiley & Sons, Ltd. Published 2013 by John Wiley & Sons Ltd.

LEARNING OUTCOMES

By the end of this chapter you should be confident and competent in working out drug dosages for neonates and paediatric patients and be aware of the relevance of body weight and body surface area when applying these calculations.

WHAT'S THE DIFFERENCE BETWEEN NURSING CALCULATIONS FOR CHILDREN AND ADULTS?

Many licensed medications have been formulated according to adult dosages, necessitating often complex calculations to administer them to neonates, children and young people. This increases the risk of miscalculation and the potential for harm. Many medications in paediatric nursing are titrated according to body weight (BW) and sometimes even according to body surface area (BSA), incorporating the patient's weight and height into the equation.

This is also true in adult nursing when dealing with very toxic medications such as chemotherapy drugs.

So, in short, there is not a lot of difference in the actual calculations between adult and paediatric nursing, but in paediatrics more emphasis is placed on certain types of calculation and fluid balance.

WORKING OUT DRUG DOSAGES

The formulas used in adult nursing fit very well in the paediatric branch of nursing, as it is the digits that are relevant when inputting these figures into the formulas.

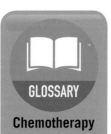

GLOSSARY

Chemotherapy drugs
Chemotherapy drugs are cell-killing drugs and growth inhibitors used in the treatment of cancer.

$$\text{Number of tablets or capsules required} = \frac{\text{what you want}}{\text{what you've got}}$$

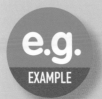

Let me show you an example...

A small child has been prescribed 100 mg of fluconazole (what you want), which comes in 50 mg capsules (what you've got). If we use the mathematical approach of 'bundling':

50 mg + 50 mg = 100 mg

we can see that two capsules are required as two lots of 50 mg make 100 mg. Or we can get used to using the formula, which will come into its own when things start to get more complicated:

$$\frac{100 \text{ mg}}{50 \text{ mg}} = 2 \text{ capsules}$$

WORKING OUT WEIGHT CONVERSIONS

We need to be absolutely confident that any dose of medication we are giving to our patient is a safe dose and for this to be achieved we often need to know the weight of our little patient and may need to undertake some conversions. Remember:

1 kg = 2.2 pounds (lb)
14 pounds (lb) = 1 stone
16 ounces (oz) = 1 pound (lb)

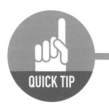

You need to know how to convert between imperial and metric units, as parents may ask for their newborn baby's weight in pounds and ounces (the imperial units) if initially given in metric units (kilograms).

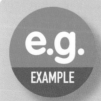

Let me show you an example...

EXAMPLE

A young child weighs 1 stone 6 lb and you need to work out the metric measure:

STEP 1: first you will need to change the weight into *pounds* by multiplying the stones by 14.

1 stone 6 lb = (1 × 14) + 6 pounds = 20 pounds in total

STEP 2: then you need to convert the pounds into kilograms by dividing by 2.2.

20 pounds/2.2 = 9.09 kg

So, the child weighs just over 9 kg.

If you need to convert metric units into imperial units, you will need to approach it this way.

A newborn baby weighs 2.8 kg and the parents want to tell their family how much the baby weighs in pounds and ounces.

STEP 1: first you will need to change the kilograms into pounds:

1 kg = 2.2 lb

2.8 kg = 2.2 × 2.8 = 6.16 lb

STEP 2: if I wanted to be more accurate, I would take the 0.16 and convert these into ounces.

1 lb = 16 oz

So, 0.16 lb × 16 oz = 2.56 oz. Therefore this little baby weighs 6 lb 3 oz (to the nearest ounce).

WORKING OUT FLUID BALANCE CALCULATIONS

Correct fluid balance calculations are vital in paediatric nursing as feeds, drug volumes and hydration fluids all need to be within the total fluid allowance of the individual baby or child for their little bodies. A typical calculation may be as follows.

Let me show you an example...

A child weighing 12 kg is prescribed 75% of maintenance fluid over 24 hours. According to local policy, 100% maintenance for a 12 kg child equates to 45 mL/hour. The child is currently receiving drugs at 5 mL/hour by continuous infusion and 10 mL of other drugs administered by injection every 8 hours. What is the amount of feed that can be given every hour?

This is how I would approach this calculation:

STEP 1: add up all the volume of drugs given per hour: 5 mL/hour + 10 mL every 8 hours. I will need to break this 10 mL up to find how much this works out in every hour: 10 mL divided by 8 hours = 1.25 mL/hour.

Total volume of drugs = 5 mL/hour + 1.25 mL/hour = 6.25 mL/hour

STEP 2: now I need to work out what 75% of 45 mL is:

$$\frac{75}{100} \times 45 = 33.75 \text{ mL}$$

This is saying that 100% = 45 mL and 75% = 33.75 mL.

STEP 3: so, now I know that 33.75 mL is the hourly fluid allowance for this child, but, minus the drugs:

33.75 mL − 6. 25 mL = 27.5 mL

Therefore, the total amount of feed that our young patient requires is 27.5 mL per hour.

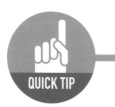

For neonatal and paediatric patients it is very important to be accurate with the volumes given.

WORKING OUT FLUID DRUG CALCULATIONS

$$\text{Volume of drug to be given} = \frac{\text{what you want}}{\text{what you've got}} \times \text{volume}$$

Again this is exactly the same formula for working out fluid doses for injection, syrups, suspensions, etc.

NOTE: remember to always check that the prescription dose and how the drug is presented are both in the same units, or you will need to convert them to the same.

Let me show you an example...

e.g.
EXAMPLE

A child is prescribed 2.5 mg orally of diazepam. It is presented as 2 mg in 5 mL of suspension. How much do you give?

$$\frac{2.5 \text{ mg}}{2 \text{ mg}} \times 5 \text{ mL} = 6.25 \text{ mL}$$

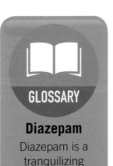

GLOSSARY

Diazepam

Diazepam is a tranquilizing muscle-relaxant drug used mainly to relieve anxiety.

DRUG DOSAGES ACCORDING TO BODY WEIGHT

Correct dosage = weight (kg) × dose

This is where we titrate the drug dose according to the baby's or child's body weight, which we addressed in Chapter 8. However, a whole dose may need to be broken down into doses to be given 2, 4, 6, 8 or 12 hours apart.

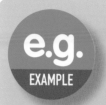

Let me show you an example...

A child weighing 29 kg has been prescribed ampicillin 80 mg/kg/day, which is to be given as four doses per day. How much do you administer in a single dose?

Using the above formula, I can work out that 29 kg × 80 mg/kg/day = 2320 mg/day. This is the amount that the child needs to receive per day, so I will need to divide this into 4 for a single dose:

2320/4 = 580 mg/dose

Therefore the child needs to receive 580 mg of the drug four times a day, as per the prescription.

DOSAGES ACCORDING TO SURFACE AREA

Body surface area (BSA) is literally the surface area of the human body. It can be worked out using an individual's height and weight measurements and may be used to calculate drug dosages and fluid intake very accurately. It is more commonly used when calculating chemotherapy doses, due to their toxicity, and in paediatric prescribing. Other influential factors when calculating BSA include the age and gender of the individual.

The most commonly used simplified formula to determine BSA is the Mosteller, which is expressed as follows:

Body surface area: the square root of product of the weight in kilograms multiplied by the height in centimetres divided by 3600. The result is in square metres.

Or how I express this:

$$\text{BSA (m}^2) = \sqrt{\frac{\text{height (cm)} \times \text{weight (kg)}}{3600}}$$

Then, to calculate BSA using this formula, I get my calculator: I put in the height (or length) of the child in centimetres and multiply it by the weight of the child in kilograms. I then divide the result by 3600 (don't worry about where the 3600 comes from, just go with it). When I have an answer I press the square root button on my calculator to get the BSA in square metres (m^2).

However, many people use a scale called a nomogram to estimate BSA, although it is considered to be much less accurate that the Mosteller formula. The figure shows a nomogram for calculating BSA in infants. There are separate nomograms for infants, children and adults.

Let me show you how to use the nomogram. First, get a ruler or something with a straight edge. If we want to find the BSA of an infant with a length of 70 cm and a weight of 32 kg we place the straight edge on the height scale at 70 cm and across to the weight scale at 32 kg. The straight edge crosses the surface area scale at approximately 0.78. This means that the BSA is 0.78 m^2.

Now, put the same details into the Mosteller formula. You will need a calculator for this exercise, one with a square root button:

$$\frac{\text{Height} \times \text{weight}}{3600} = \frac{70 \text{ cm} \times 32 \text{ kg}}{3600} =$$

Using your calculator, input:

$$70 \times 32 = 2240/3600 = 0.62$$

Then find the square root, or press the square root button on your calculator, and you get 0.79 m^2.

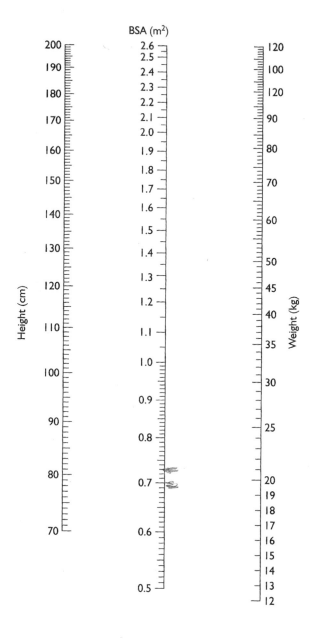

BSA (m²)

Height (cm)

Weight (kg)

ACTIVITY

Activity 12.1

Now, let's put everything into practice and try a few questions. If you get stuck, just go back to the section dealing with that particular question and follow the steps again. All the answers, with the workings out, are given in the Answers section at the end of the book. Don't peep: have a go first!

1 Oral paracetamol 50 mg is prescribed. It is presented as 120 mg in 5 mL. What volume do you draw up?

2 Oral phenobarbital (phenobarbitone) 35 mg is prescribed. It is available as 15 mg in 5 mL. What volume would you give?

3 Erythromycin 30 mg/kg/day is prescribed to a child weighing 12 kg. The child is to receive this medication over four doses per day. Calculate a single dose.

4 A child weighing 36 kg has been prescribed flucloxacillin 80 mg/kg/day over four doses. Calculate a single dose.

5 A child weighs 2 stone 8 lb. Work out the metric weight.

6 A child weighs 6.10 kg. Work out the imperial weight.

7 A child weighs 12 kg and is prescribed 75% of maintenance fluid over 24 hours (100% maintenance for a 12 kg child is 45 mL/hour). The child is presently receiving medication by continuous infusion at 2 mL/hour, 8 mL of another medication every 8 hours and 2 mL of a third drug every 6 hours. What is the amount of feed that this child can receive every hour?

8 Digoxin 125 micrograms is prescribed. The drug is presented as 0.5 mg in 2 mL. Calculate the volume you need to draw up.

9 Pethidine 20 mg is prescribed. The drug is presented as 50 mg in 1 mL. Calculate the volume to be drawn up.

10 Use the nomogram shown in this chapter to find the body surface area (BSA) of a child weighing 16.0 kg with a length of 94 cm.

11 Use the nomogram to find the BSA of a child with a length of 95 cm and a weight of 14.0 kg.

12 Using the Mosteller formula, work out the BSA of a child weighing 14.0 kg and with a length of 87 cm.

KEY POINTS

- Understanding weight conversions.
- Understanding fluid balance calculations.
- Looking at the calculation of body surface area using a nomogram.
- Looking at the calculation of body surface area using the Mosteller formula.

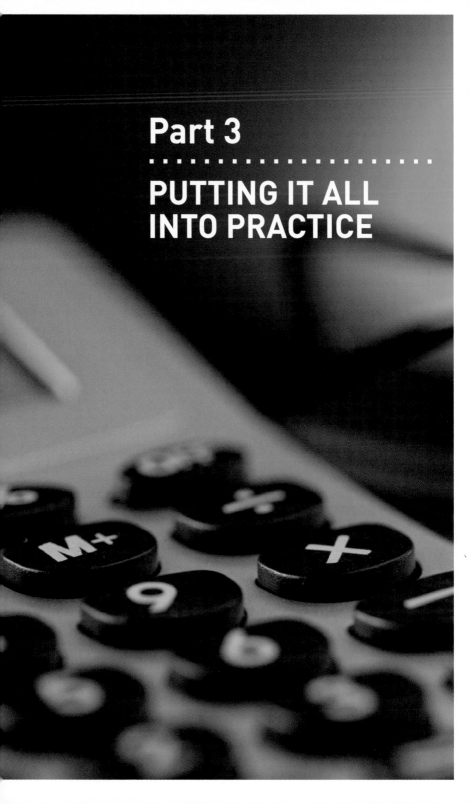

Part 3

PUTTING IT ALL INTO PRACTICE

Chapter 13
FLUID CHARTS

Calculation Skills for Nurses, First Edition. Claire Boyd
© 2013 John Wiley & Sons, Ltd. Published 2013 by John Wiley & Sons Ltd.

LEARNING OUTCOMES

By the end of this chapter you should have a working knowledge of fluid charts and the importance of fluid balance.

A fluid chart is a record of the amount of fluids a patient has taken in during a day (i.e. drinks and any other fluids, such as 5% dextrose saline via the IV route) and the patient's fluid output (i.e. urine, vomit, etc.). The output total is subtracted from the intake total and the balance is recorded. When intake is greater than output a positive balance is recorded, but if intake is less than output the fluid balance is recorded as being negative.

Accurately monitoring a patient's fluid balance is crucial to a patient's well-being, as the body works within very narrow parameters and is always striving for homeostasis. In short, any water loss needs to be replaced for the body's water volume to remain constant.

In males, total body fluid constitutes approximately 60% of the body weight. In females, total body fluid constitutes approximately 52% of total body weight.

Too little fluid in the body, perhaps due to excessive diarrhoea, vomiting or sweating due to fever, is known as hypovalemia. Too much fluid, perhaps caused by over-infusion of intravenous fluids, congestive cardiac failure or renal failure, is known as hypervalemia. It takes just a small amount of variation from the norm to cause havoc within the body:

- a reduction of 5% causes thirst,
- a reduction of 8% causes illness,
- a reduction of 10% can cause death.

Let me show you an example...

Here's how to work out a person's fluid balance.
Today I have drunk:

- two cups of coffee: 150 mL per cup,
- four cups of tea: 150 mL per cup,
- one cola: 300 mL,
- one bottle of spring water: 500 mL.

I add all this up, which equals 1700 mL. This is my input.

I went to the toilet to pass urine four times throughout the day, passing 400 mL, 600 mL, 200 mL and 450 mL. I add this up, which equals 1650 mL. This is my output.

I then subtract my output from my input = 1700 mL − 1650 mL = 50 mL. This is my fluid balance, pretty good! Note that we tend to look at longer periods to see trends for fluid balance.

Fluid balance

Fluid balance relates to the difference between the amount of fluid taken into the body and the amount excreted or lost.

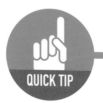

The 24-hour fluid record chart generally starts at 08.00 and the final tally gets totted up at 07:00, just before the early shift for the day.

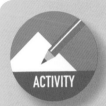

Activity 13.1

ACTIVITY

Mrs Maxwell has had a cup of tea (150 mL) at the following times:

08:00	150 mL
10:00	150 mL
12:00	150 mL
14:00	150 mL
18:00	150 mL
22:00	150 mL

Mrs Maxwell has also had a blackcurrant drink (188 mL) at 13:00 and a small cola (150 mL) at 17:00. Finally, at 06:00 Mrs Maxwell drank 1500 mL of water from her water jug.

Mrs Maxwell has a urinary catheter in place which was emptied at 16:00; the amount was 750 mL.

Plot all these amounts on the input part of the fluid balance chart (see Appendix 1).

What is Mrs Maxwell's fluid balance? (That's input amount *minus* output amount.)

Activity 13.2

ACTIVITY

Work out the total input, total output and fluid balance for these patients.

1 Intake
IV fluid = 1500 mL
oral fluids = 75 mL
Output
urine = 1020 mL
vomit = 75 mL
wound drainage = 15 mL

2 Intake
IV fluid = 850 mL
oral fluids = 275 mL
Output
urine = 525 mL
vomit = 60 mL
wound drainage = 50 mL

3 Intake
oral fluids = 950 mL
Output
urine = 500 mL
liquid diarrhoea = 400 mL

4 Intake
oral fluids = 1750 mL
Output
urine = 500 mL

5 Intake
IV fluids = 1 L
oral fluids = 150 mL
Output
vomit = 50 mL
wound leak = 50 mL

6 Intake
oral fluids = 500 mL
Output
urine = 900 mL

KEY POINTS

- Looking at fluid charts.
- Looking at fluid balance.

Chapter 14
. . . .
MALNUTRITION UNIVERSAL SCREENING TOOL (MUST) ASSESSMENT

Calculation Skills for Nurses, First Edition. Claire Boyd
© 2013 John Wiley & Sons, Ltd. Published 2013 by John Wiley & Sons Ltd.

LEARNING OUTCOMES

By the end of this chapter you should have a working knowledge of the Malnutrition Universal Screening Tool (MUST) assessment.

MUST, or Malnutrition Universal Screening Tool, is a five-step screening tool to identify *adults* (not children) who are malnourished, at risk of malnutrition (undernutrition) or obese. It also includes management guidelines which can be used to develop a care plan. Take a few minutes to look at the MUST assessment guidelines in Appendix 2.

Now let me show you how to use the MUST assessment by working through the steps.

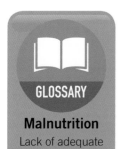

GLOSSARY

Malnutrition
Lack of adequate nutrition.

Malnourished
Suffering from malnutrition.

Obese
Excess body fat or overweight.

Step 1 First I work out the body mass index (BMI) of my patient, in this case a gentleman who measures 1.76 m in height and weighs 95 kg. Using these figures on the chart, I find that this equates to a BMI of 31 kg/m^2, and score of zero.

Step 2 I look to see if there has been any unplanned weight loss in the past 3–6 months. There is none for my make-believe patient, so the score is another zero.

Step 3 For this part of the process I look to see if there are any acute diseases present, and as there are none for my patient, the score is zero.

Step 4 This next part requires me to add up all my scores to establish the overall risk of malnutrition and, as I have a zero, the MUST score is deemed to be low risk and so I follow the management guidelines for low-risk patients.

Note: even though this make-believe patient is obese, this does not rule him out from malnutrition. He may be big, but his diet may be very poor nutritionally.

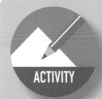

Activity 14.1

ACTIVITY

Work through the five MUST steps.

Step 1   Dennis Langley is 85 years old. He is 5 feet 5 inches in height and weighs 85 kg. What is his BMI score, and his MUST score for Step 1?

Step 2   Four months ago, Dennis' wife died and he lost some weight, but less than 5%. What is his MUST score for Step 2?

Step 3   Dennis has stopped eating and is drinking very little: this has got worse over the last 5 days. What is his MUST score or Step 3?

Step 4   What is his overall risk of malnutrition score?

Step 5   What is his management strategy?

KEY POINT

- How to use the Malnutrition Universal Screening Tool (MUST) to identify adults who are malnourished, at risk of malnutrition or obese.

Chapter 15

. . . .

EARLY WARNING SCORE (EWS) ASSESSMENT

Calculation Skills for Nurses, First Edition. Claire Boyd
© 2013 John Wiley & Sons, Ltd. Published 2013 by John Wiley & Sons Ltd.

LEARNING OUTCOMES

By the end of this chapter you should have a working knowledge of the Early Warning Score (EWS) assessment.

Early Warning Scores (EWSs) are used to assess patients using a physiological scoring system, taken from bedside observations, and plotted on a Bristol Observation Chart. Each observation generates a score, which is explained in the table.

Score	Nursing Action
0–1	Continue with routine observations.
2–3	Inform the nurse in charge. Increase frequency of observations to hourly.
≥4	Contact the medical team urgently. Patient to be reviewed within 15 minutes. Inform nurse in charge. Increase the frequency of observations to half hourly. Complete a report of action.

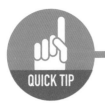

QUICK TIP

A score of 4 or more with the EWS assessment indicates cause for concern, initiating immediate action by a call for medical assistance.

The observations assessed are the patient's respiratory rate, *systolic* blood pressure, heart rate, temperature, oxygen saturation range (SpO$_2$) and mental response using the AVPU system. This is an assessment of consciousness, stating whether the patient is **a**lert, responding to **v**erbal or **p**ain stimuli, or **u**nresponsive (which is where the acronym AVPU comes from). So, in short, the EWS can alert us to the fact that a patient is deteriorating, necessitating medical assistance to be sought and facilitating a more favourable outcome for the patient in the majority of cases: the EWS saves lives!

Target oxygen saturation ranges are shown in this table.

94–98%	92–98%	88–92%
Age <70 years	Age >70 years	Risk factors present

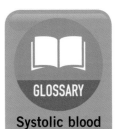

GLOSSARY

Systolic blood pressure

The systolic blood pressure is the pressure exerted on the arterial walls due to the contraction of the heart.

- Administer oxygen to achieve saturation in the prescribed range.
- Only administer oxygen if it is prescribed, except in an emergency when oxygen may be given and actions recorded in medical notes later.
- **Increase** oxygen dose if saturation below range.
- **Decrease** oxygen dose or stop supplementary oxygen if saturation exceeds target range. High levels of oxygen are harmful to some patients.

The EWS assessment can be used in conjunction with the Early Patient Assessment and Response assessment (known as EPAR), or the ABCDE.

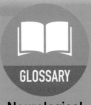

GLOSSARY

Neurological observation

A neurological observation is a collection of information in regard to the central nervous system (the brain and spinal cord).

A Airway

B Breathing

C Circulation (also think about cannulation for peripheral access in an emergency)

D Disability (includes neurological observations, diuresis, drugs and diabetes, i.e. monitoring blood glucose). If the AVPU assessment falls, then a full Glasgow Coma Scale assessment will need to be performed.

E Exposure (looking for bleeding/areas of concern on the body) and Early call for help.

Let me show you how to use the EWS using the Bristol Observation Chart (which is shown in Appendix 3).

- First I obtain my patient's respiratory rate, which on this occasion is 32 breaths per minute, which generates a score of 2 points.

- Then I look at my patient's oxygen levels and see if the oxygen is within the prescribed levels on the prescription chart. If my make-believe patient had an oxygen level reading of 91% and this was out of the prescribed range, this would necessitate a score of 1.
- My patient's blood pressure is 198/92 mmHg. The systolic part of this reading (198 mmHg) does not generate a score on the Bristol Observation Chart.
- Then I look at the heart rate, which at 102 beats per minute generates a score of 1 point.
- The neurological response is Alert, and does not generate a score.
- The temperature is 37.9°C, which again does not generate a score.
- Next I add up the scores: 2 + 1 + 0 + 1 + 0 + 0 = 4. As 4 is the trigger score, I would contact a medic immediately and call for assistance.

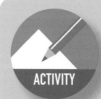

Activity 15.1

Using the Bristol Observation Chart shown in Appendix 3, work out the EWS for Mrs Eunice Yonder.

1   Eunice is 62 years old and has been admitted to hospital due to shortness of breath and difficulty breathing. Her observations on admittance are:
Respiratory rate: 30 breaths per minute (bpm)
SpO$_2$: 92% on air
Blood pressure: 165/80 mmHg
Heart rate: 90 beats per minute
AVPU: Alert
Temperature: 37.9°C
What is her EWS?

2   One hour later, you notice Eunice appears confused and less responsive.
    After performing a blood glucose test, which are within normal parameters,
    you perform another set of observations:
    Respiratory rate: 35 breaths per minute
    SpO_2: 89% on air
    Blood pressure: 180/80 mmHg
    Heart rate: 140 beats per minute
    AVPU: Verbal
    Temperature: 38.2°C
    What is her latest EWS?

KEY POINTS

- How to use the Early Warning Score (EWS) tool.
- Understanding the AVPU assessment.

Chapter 16

WATERLOW ASSESSMENT

Calculation Skills for Nurses, First Edition. Claire Boyd
© 2013 John Wiley & Sons, Ltd. Published 2013 by John Wiley & Sons Ltd.

LEARNING OUTCOMES

By the end of this chapter you should have a working knowledge of the Waterlow risk assessment tool.

The Waterlow Pressure Ulcer Prevention/Treatment Policy, or Waterlow risk assessment tool (see Appendix 4), helps us to establish an individual's risk factors for acquiring a pressure ulcer. This forewarns us of the need to utilise specialised equipment such as pressure-relieving mattresses on a patient's bed, and other devices such as cushions and heel guards. The Waterlow tool looks at a patient's medical state, age and gender to work out this score.

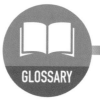

GLOSSARY

Pressure ulcer

A pressure ulcer is an area of skin that has broken down after constant pressure has been applied, or in a combination with shear and/or friction.

e.g.

EXAMPLE

Let me show you an example...

Let me show you how to use the Waterlow assessment tool, using the form shown in Appendix 4.

- I always start off with the age and gender of the patient (don't ask me why, I just do!). So, if I had a male patient this would mean a score of 1 point. If he were aged 72, this would be 3 points. Therefore, in this section (Sex/Age) my patient has scored 4 points for his age and gender.

- Then I go to the start of the assessment tool, to the Build/Weight section and input the details: my patient has an average body mass index, scoring 0 points.
- The next section is the Skin Type and I can see that my patient is quite oedematous or, as he himself describes, 'puffy', so I score him 1 point.
- I have already completed the Sex/Age section, so I move on to the Nutrition section. As my patient has not lost weight recently I move on to Section C and I learn that my patient has presently lost his appetite, so I score him 1 point.
- I then move on to the Continence section and as my patient has no issues in this area, he gets a score of 0 points.
- The next section I look at is Mobility. He has back pain and this is restricting his mobility, necessitating long periods sitting in a chair; I score him a 3.
- Lastly I look at Special Risks and as he is a smoker he gets 1 point and he has an Hb value of 4, so he gets 2 points. He is also on high-dose steroids and anti-inflammatory medication for his back pain, for which he gets a further score of 4 points.
- Now I add up the score: $1 + 3 + 0 + 1 + 1 + 0 + 3 + 1 + 2 + 4 = 16$, which equates to a high risk of getting pressure ulcers.

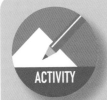

Activity 16.1

ACTIVITY

Using the Waterlow risk assessment tool, work out Molly's Waterlow score. This is done by gathering all the information we have to hand and giving it a score against the assessment tool. For example, Molly immediately gets 2 points just for being female.

Molly Jeffreys is 70 years old and is usually average weight/build for her height. She has, however, recently lost 9.5 kg in weight, due to 'going off' her food.

Molly has very thin skin, with a lack of subcutaneous tissue. Daisy states that she feels 'very weak' and her mobility is restricted because of this.

After a review by her GP, Molly was found to have a urinary tract infection (and is now wearing a pad and pants due to some urinary incontinence), and also has anaemia.

What is Molly's Waterlow score?

KEY POINT

- How to use the Waterlow risk assessment tool for pressure ulcers.

Chapter 17
. . . .
PRESCRIPTION CHARTS

Calculation Skills for Nurses, First Edition. Claire Boyd
© 2013 John Wiley & Sons, Ltd. Published 2013 by John Wiley & Sons Ltd.

LEARNING OUTCOMES

By the end of this chapter you should have working knowledge of a prescription chart.

Remember that a prescription chart is a legal document, and that to work out how many tablets or capsules, or millilitres of fluid, that we need to administer we use the following formulas.

For tablets or capsules:

$$\text{Number of tablets or capsules required} = \frac{\text{what you want}}{\text{what you've got}}$$

For a liquid:

$$\text{Volume of drug to be given} = \frac{\text{what you want}}{\text{what you've got}} \times \text{volume}$$

So, if a medic has prescribed 60 mg of codeine phosphate to a child, every 4–6 hours (maximum dose of 240 mg daily), and the drug is presented in 30 mg tablets, this works out as:

$$\frac{60 \text{ mg}}{30 \text{ mg}} = 2 \text{ tablets}$$

Activity 17.1

Look at the prescription chart and for the drugs listed work out how many tablets, capsules or millilitres of injection the patient requires each dose, and any special considerations you need to consider. The available formulations of the drugs are given below.

NOTE: when administering drugs, the nurse is required to know about the drug itself (any contra-indications, etc.), and you may wish to use a copy of the British National Formulary while undertaking this activity.

1   Erythromycin: on hand are 250 mg tablets.
2   Aspirin (dispersible tablets): on hand are 75 mg tablets.
3   Tramadol hydrochloride: on hand are 50 mg/mL ampoules for intravenous injection.
4   Propranolol hydrochloride: on hand are 160 mg capsules.
5   Hydroxocobalamin intramuscular injection: on hand are 1 mg/1 mL ampoules.
6   Ketorolac trometamol: on hand are 10 mg/mL ampoules for intravenous injection.

GLOSSARY

Contra-indication
A condition that makes a particular treatment or procedure inadvisable.

6 hourly	06.00–12.00–18.00–24.00	SURNAME (MR/MRS/MISS)		DATE OF BIRTH	UNIT NUMBER
8 hourly	06.00–14.00–22.00	FIRST NAMES		SEX	CONSULTANT
12 hourly	09.00–21.00	ADDRESS			

REGULAR PRESCRIPTIONS

	Date	Drug	Dose	Route	Times of Administration	Other Directions	Doctor's	Date	Pharm

REGULAR PRESCRIPTIONS

	Date	Drug (approved name – BLOCK CAPITALS)	Dose	Route	6	12	18	24	Other Directions Duration	Doctor's Signature	Date	Pharm
1	TODAY	ERYTHROMYCIN	500 MG	O	√	√	√	√		A Doctor		
2	TODAY	ASPIRIN (DISPERSIBLE)	300 MG	O		√			AFTER FOOD	A Doctor		
3	TODAY	TRAMADOL HYDROCHLORIDE	75 MG	IV	√	√	√	√	GIVE OVER 2–3 MINS	A Doctor		
4	TODAY	PROPRANOLOL	80 MG	O	√		√			A Doctor		
5	TODAY	HYDROXOCOBALAMIN	1 MG	IM	√				GIVE EVERY 3 MONTHS	A Doctor		
6	TODAY	KETOROLAC TROMETAMOL	35 MG	IV	√		√		ADMINISTER OVER >15 SECONDS	A Doctor		
7												
8												
9												
10												
11												
12												
13												
14												
15												

AS REQUIRED PRESCRIPTIONS

	Date	Drug (approved name – BLOCK CAPITALS)	Dose	Route	Directions	Maximum Frequency	Doctor's Signature	Date	Pharm
1									
2									
3									
4									
5									
6									
7									
8									
9									

Source: Prescription chart. Reproduced here with permission from North Bristol NHS Trust and University Hospitals Bristol NHS Foundation Trust.

Activity 17.2

A patient's prescription chart shows that the patient is prescribed:

1   soluble aspirin 150 mg,
2   diazepam 12.5 mg,
3   digoxin 125 micrograms,
4   paracetamol 1 gram,
5   atenolol 75 mg,
6   furosemide 40 mg.

Below are the labels on the bottles in the drug trolley, which have all been mixed up. Can you work out the number of tablets or capsules to be administered in each case?

Digoxin **0.25 mg**	**Soluble aspirin** **300 mg**	**Diazepam** **5 mg**
Paracetamol **500 mg**	**Furosemide** **40 mg**	**Atenolol** **50 mg**

KEY POINT

- Administering medications according to a patient's prescription chart.

Chapter 18
. . . .
LOOKING AT
BUDGETS

Calculation Skills for Nurses, First Edition. Claire Boyd
© 2013 John Wiley & Sons, Ltd. Published 2013 by John Wiley & Sons Ltd.

LEARNING OUTCOMES

By the end of this chapter you should have a working knowledge of calculating simple budgets and reading simple charts.

In health care, applying mathematics takes many different forms. For example, just knowing that on one ward in a directorate in the hospital they employ five band 6 nurses, all on approximately £32 000 per annum, I know that their annual salaries amount to 6 × £32 000, or £192 000. See if you can work out the training budget for the care home described below.

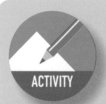

Activity 18.1

ACTIVITY

A care home has a budget of £2200 per year for training. The manager would like the home's registered general nurses to have training in venepuncture and adult male catheterisation, which can be received from the local NHS Trust. She would also like the care assistants in the home to undertake training in catheter care.

This year, half of the care assistant staff are due for their Basic Clinical Skills 2-yearly update, again provided by the local NHS Trust.

1   Look at the staff numbers and cost sheet below and state how much this training will cost. Does the care home have enough money to pay for it?

Job title	Number of staff
Registered general nurses	6
Care assistants	24
Customer services	12

Training session	Cost
Venepuncture	£57.50 per person
Adult male urinary catheterisation	£57.50 per person
Catheter care	£57.50 per person
Basic Clinical Skills	£400 per session (no more than 12 individuals in each session)

2   What is the ratio of registered general nurses to care assistants to customer services staff?

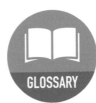

GLOSSARY

Venepuncture
Venepuncture is when a vein is punctured to obtain blood as part of a medical procedure.

In health care, you will also be expected to interpret data.

The chart shows the UK Central Government expenditure for public sector departments in 2009–2010. The revenue to pay for this expenditure is gathered by Her Majesty's Revenue and Customs in the form of taxes.

Expenditure (£, bn)

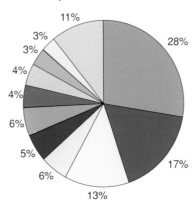

- Social Protection
- Health
- Education
- Defence
- Public Order and Safety
- Debt interest
- Housing and environment
- Personal social services
- Transport
- Industry, Agriculture & Employment
- Other

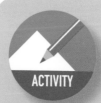

Activity 18.2

Looking at the UK Government expenditure chart, answer these questions.
1. How much is spent on health care?
2. What is the largest expenditure?
3. How much is spent on housing and environment?
4. What is the financial difference between health, and housing and environment?

KEY POINTS

- Looking at budgets.
- How to interpret data.

Chapter 19

INTERPRETING DATA

Calculation Skills for Nurses, First Edition. Claire Boyd

© 2013 John Wiley & Sons, Ltd. Published 2013 by John Wiley & Sons Ltd.

LEARNING OUTCOMES

By the end of this chapter you should have a working knowledge of interpreting basic data.

I would like to know how many patients receiving a blood transfusion had an incident involving a transfusion-related acute lung injury. I look at the pie chart showing the incidences of serious hazards in transfusion. First I need to find out how transfusion-related acute lung injury is expressed, see I look at the key and see that it is shown as TRALI. Then I look for this on the chart and can see that 15 patients, or 1.0% of the sample, experienced this reaction.

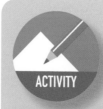

Activity 19.1

The pie chart shows the Serious Hazards of (Blood) Transfusion audit for the year 2010 in an NHS Trust, a snapshot of this time.

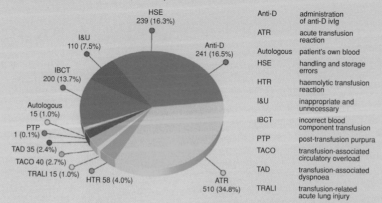

Serious Hazards of (Blood) Transfusion audit, showing numbers of cases in 2010.

Source: Knowles, S. (ed.) and Cohen, H. on behalf of the Serious Hazards of Transfusion (SHOT) Steering Group (2011) *Serious Hazards of Transfusion (SHOT) Report 2010.*

Dyspnoea

Dyspnoea means a difficulty breathing.

Post-transfusion purpura

An adverse reaction to a blood transfusion causing a rash or redness.

GLOSSARY

1 Where are the most hazards occurring?
2 Where are the fewest hazards occurring?

Blood glucose, sodium, potassium and other blood electrolytes are measured in millimoles or micromoles per litre of blood. This is how biochemistry results are presented.

A mole is the molecular weight of a substance in grams.

1 mole contains 1000 millimoles (mmol)
1 millimole contains 1000 micromoles (μmol)

QUICK TIP

As a nurse you may see μ in laboratory test results: this means 'micro'. So, μmol means micromoles.

Let me show you an example...

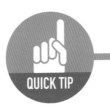

EXAMPLE

A patient's laboratory results have just been returned. Patient A has a result of urea at 5.5 mmol/L. Let's look at the table of the safe ranges for blood electrolytes and other substances. The acceptable range for urea is 2.5–7.8 mmol/L, so this patient's urea is not a cause for concern.

Test name	Units	Range	
		Low	High
Sodium	mmol/L	133	146
Potassium	mmol/L	3.5	5.3
Urea	mmol/L	2.5	7.8
Chloride	mmol/L	95	108
Bicarbonate	mmol/L	22	29
Phosphate	mmol/L	0.8	1.5
Magnesium	mmol/L	0.7	1.0
Osmolality	mmol/kg	275	295
Alkaline phosphatase (ALP)	units, U/L	30	130
Creatine kinase (CK)	units, U/L	40 25	320 (M) 200 (F)
Bilirubin (total)	μmol/L		<21
Adjusted calcium	mmol/L	2.2	2.6
Urate	μmol/L	200 140	430 (M) 360 (F)
Carbamazepine	mg/L	4	12
Phenobarbitone	mg/L	10	40
Phenytoin	mg/L	5	20
Lithium	mmol/L	0.4	1.0
24 h urine urate	mmol/24 h	1.5	4.5
24 h urine phosphate	mmol/24 h	15	50
24 h urine magnesium	mmol/24 h	2.4	6.5

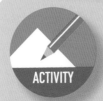

Activity 19.2

Patient B's results have just been returned. Here they are:

Sodium	**145 mmol/L**
Bicarbonate	**30 mmol/L**

Looking at the table, are these results within the acceptable range?

KEY POINTS

- Looking at biochemistry results.
- Looking at the moles, millimoles and micromoles.

Chapter 20
. . . .
EMPLOYMENT SERVICES

Calculation Skills for Nurses, First Edition. Claire Boyd
© 2013 John Wiley & Sons, Ltd. Published 2013 by John Wiley & Sons Ltd.

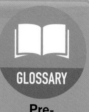

LEARNING OUTCOMES

By the end of this chapter you should be competent in
answering a pre-employment calculations test.

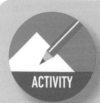

GLOSSARY

Pre-employment calculations test

A test used
to determine
competence in
maths skills.

Many healthcare employers now include a test of
calculations competence at the interview stage. Talk about
added pressure! This chapter gives an example of sample
questions in actual test papers. Some employers allow
calculators, but others may not, and pass rates are variable
from trust to trust. For example, 60% may be the pass rate
at one trust, 100% may be the pass rate at another. You
may wish to gather your formula sheet for this exercise, as
some trusts may include these at the start of the paper but,
again, others may not.

Now, let's see how you do answering the questions in this
sample test paper, Activity 20.1. You may not use a calculator.
The activity is designed to assess your ability to calculate
doses from a prescription. The process of calculating doses
is the same regardless of the drug prescribed, or the age,
clinical setting or diagnosis of the patient.

Activity 20.1

ACTIVITY

NOTE: you have 1 hour to complete this test.

1   Gentamicin is dispensed as 80 mg in 2 mL. The prescription is to
     administer 50 mg of gentamicin. What volume of gentamicin do you
     administer?
2   IV metronidazole 500 mg is dispensed in a 100 mL bag. A child is
     prescribed 300 mg of metronidazole. What volume do you administer?
3   A patient is prescribed 60 mg of codeine phosphate. The drug is
     presented in tablets of 30 mg. How many tablets does the patient require?

4 Paracetamol is prescribed as 10 mg/kg and needs to be given 8 hourly. How much would you give to a baby weighing 2.5 kg?

5 1000 mL of sodium chloride 0.9% is prescribed to run over 12 hours. Calculate the drip rate in drops per minute.

6 Heparin is dispensed as 25 000 units in 5 mL. 30 000 units of heparin is prescribed, to be diluted to 48 mL.
   (a) What volume of heparin would you administer?
   (b) How much dilutant is required?

7 A woman has been prescribed 450 mL of blood, to run over 4 hours. Calculate the drip rate per minute using a filtered-blood administration set.

8 600 mL of fluid is dripping at 20 drops per minute. The IV set delivers 15 drops/mL. How long will the infusion take?

9 Hydrocortisone is dispensed as 100 mg in 2 mL. The patient is prescribed 75 mg of hydrocortisone. What volume of the drug would you administer?

10 A patient is prescribed 225 mg of ranitidine. Each tablet contains 150 mg. How many tablets does the patient require?

KEY POINT

- Looking at how to answer a pre-employment test paper correctly.

Chapter 21

. . . .

BODY MASS INDEX

Calculation Skills for Nurses, First Edition. Claire Boyd

© 2013 John Wiley & Sons, Ltd. Published 2013 by John Wiley & Sons Ltd.

LEARNING OUTCOMES

By the end of this chapter you will have the knowledge to work out a patient's body mass index (BMI).

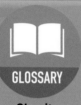

GLOSSARY

Obesity

Having excess body fat. For adults 35 years of age and older, having a BMI greater than 30 kg/m^2 is considered obese.

Underweight

A BMI of under 18.5 kg/m^2 in adults.

Many care homes and institutions use the Malnutrition Universal Screening Tool (MUST) to identify malnourished or obese adult patients/service users, and the body mass index (BMI) chart is part of this assessment tool. Although we looked at this in Chapter 14, we still need to know what a body mass index means and how to obtain this figure. The MUST is shown in Appendix 2.

BMI is actually a number that has been calculated by dividing your weight in kilograms by your height in square metres. Often height is measured in centimetres, so we need to divide this figure by 100 to obtain the height in metres.

$$BMI = \text{weight (kg)/height (m}^2)$$

The BMI value is an indicator of body fatness for most people and is a useful tool in determining obesity or identifying adults who are underweight, which may be a health risk.

BMI GUIDELINES

Underweight	BMI <18.4 kg/m^2
Acceptable	BMI 18.5–24.9 kg/m^2
Overweight	BMI 25–29.9 kg/m^2
Obese	BMI 30–39.9 kg/m^2
Morbidly obese	BMI >40 kg/m^2

A healthy BMI value for most adults is between 18.5 and 24.9 kg/m^2.

Although the BMI does compare well with body fatness for most people, it is not a definite indicator of a percentage of an individual's body fat. The correlation between body fat and BMI also has some variables:

- women tend to have more body fat than men at the same BMI,
- older people, on average, tend to have more body fat than younger adults at the same BMI,
- athletes have a high BMI due to their increased muscularity rather than increased body fatness.

Let me show you how I would work out the BMI for an individual:

Height: 185 cm
Weight: 91 kg

$$BMI = weight\ (kg)/height\ (m^2)$$

First change the height in centimetres to metres = 185/100 = 1.85 metres.

Then square the 1.85 = 1.85 × 1.85 = 3.4225.

Then use the formula:

$$\frac{91}{3.4} = 26.76 = 27\ kg/m^2$$

Oops! This person falls into the category of being overweight, which raises their risk of premature death.

Activity 21.1

ACTIVITY

Patient A weighs 105 kg and is 1.65 m in height. Using the steps above find out the patient's BMI.

Activity 21.2

Find out your height in metres and your weight in kilograms. Then, using the steps above, find out your BMI.

KEY POINT

- **How to work out an adult's body mass index.**

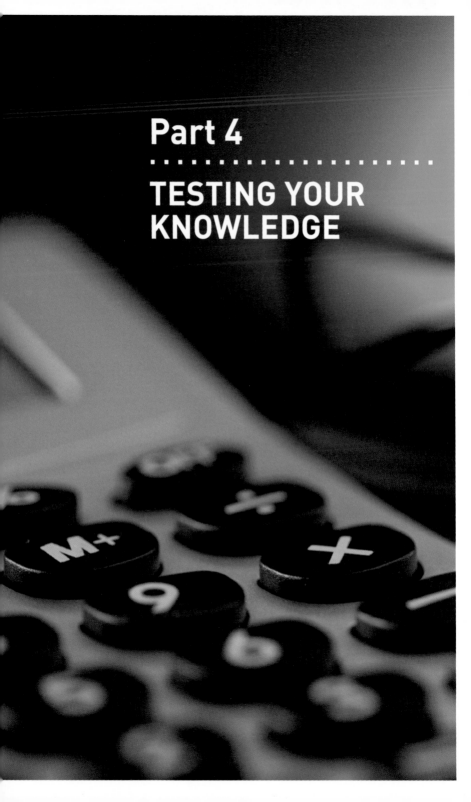

Part 4

TESTING YOUR KNOWLEDGE

Chapter 22
. . . .
KNOWLEDGE TESTS

Calculation Skills for Nurses, First Edition. Claire Boyd
© 2013 John Wiley & Sons, Ltd. Published 2013 by John Wiley & Sons Ltd.

These knowledge tests have been compiled to test your knowledge of everything we have looked at throughout the book, and to show you the calculation problems you may come across in your healthcare career.

KNOWLEDGE TEST 1

1   Waterlow Pressure Ulcer Prevention/Treatment: Walter Jones is an 80-year-old male with a BMI of 20 kg/m^2. Walter has oedematous legs and has Type 2 diabetes. Walter has a good appetite. Presently he has been restricted in his mobility due to his swollen legs. What is Walter's Waterlow score?

2   Early Warning Score (EWS): Jane Fielding has the following observations:

Respiratory rate	18 breaths per minute
SpO$_2$	99% on air
Blood pressure	130/80 mmHg
Heart rate	80 beats per minute
Neurological response	Alert

What is her EWS score?

3   A patient has been prescribed 35 mg of codeine phosphate by injection. Ampoules of 60 mg in 1 mL are available. How many millilitres will you administer?

4   A patient is prescribed 27 mg of Adenocor. Stock ampoules contain 30 mg in 10 mL. What volume of drug needs to be administered?

5   A drug is presented as 4 g in 400 mL. A patient weighing 100 kg is prescribed 10 mg/kg/h of the drug.
    (a) How many milligrams per hour of the drug does the patient need?
    (b) How many millilitres per hour do you set the infusion pump at?

6   Furosemide is available in a concentration of 20 mg in 2 mL. A patient is prescribed 15 mg intravenously as

a bolus. It is to be given at a maximum rate of 3 mg/minute.

(a) What volume of furosemide would you administer?

(b) How many minutes should it be given over?

7 IV morphine sulphate comes as 15 mg in 1 mL. The prescription is to administer 6 mg of morphine sulphate. What volume of the drug would you administer?

8 Amoxicillin is presented as 500 mg per ampoule. It is to be diluted to a volume of 10 mL. Your patient is prescribed 1.5 g. What volume of amoxicillin do you draw up?

9 Caffeine base is prescribed at 2.5 mg/kg per 24 hours. The patient, a baby, weighs 1.2 kg.

(a) What amount of caffeine base is prescribed?

(b) Caffeine base comes as 5 mg in 1 mL. This needs to be reconstituted five times with 0.9% sodium chloride (NaCl) and infused over 10 minutes. What is the total volume to be infused?

10 Benzylpenicillin IV is prescribed to a baby as 50 mg/kg. The baby weighs 3.4 kg.

(a) What dose is prescribed?

(b) The drug comes as 600 mg in 4 mL of water. How much do you give?

KNOWLEDGE TEST 2

1 Malnutrition Universal Screening Tool (MUST): Max Norman is a 52-year-old gentleman. He is 5 feet 8½ inches in height and weighs 100 kg. What is his BMI?

2 Early Warning Score (EWS): Robert Hayes has the following observations:

Respiratory rate	36 breaths per minute
SpO_2	89% on air
Blood pressure	108/70 mmHg
Heart rate	129 beats per minute
Neurological response	Alert

What is his EWS score?

3 A patient has been prescribed 75 mg of pethidine by injection. 50 mg in 1 mL of liquid for injection is available. How many millilitres will you administer?

4 A patient is prescribed 75 micrograms of fenatyl citrate intravenously. 0.1 mg in 1 mL of liquid for IV injection is available. How many millilitres will you administer?

5 Digoxin ampoules contain 500 micrograms in 2 mL. What volume is needed for an injection of 275 micrograms?

6 Ampoules of adrenaline for anaphylactic shock contain 1 mg in 1 mL (1:1000). What volume is needed for an IM injection of 500 micrograms?

7 Ampicillin 80 mg/kg per day is prescribed for a 90 kg man. The drug is to be given 6 hourly. Calculate the amount needed for a single dose.

8 Benzylpenicillin IV is prescribed as 50 mg/kg. The patient, a baby, weighs 4.2 kg.
   (a) What dose is prescribed?
   (b) The drug comes as 600 mg in 4 mL of water. How much do you give?

9 A patient is to have 2 L of clear fluids in 24 hours. He has received 700 mL in 10 hours. How many drops per minute are required to correct the infusion?

10 An insulin infusion containing 50 units of human Actrapid has been diluted with 50 mL of sodium chloride, which has been running at:

> 3 mL/hour for 1 hour
>
> 3.5 mL/hour for 2 hours
>
> 2 mL/hour for 2 hours
>
> 2.5 mL/hour for 2 hours
>
> 4 mL/hour for 1 hour

How many units of Actrapid insulin in total has the patient received?

KNOWLEDGE TEST 3

1   Waterlow Pressure Ulcer Prevention/Treatment: Violet Simms is a 90-year-old lady with a BMI of 18 kg/m^2. Violet is covered in bruises due to falls, and has 'tissue paper' skin. Violet has gone off her food lately and is eating very poorly, causing her to lose approximately 1.8 kg in the last few weeks. Violet has been experiencing some urinary incontinence recently and has just been found to be suffering from a high temperature. Violet is reluctant to mobilise independently since her falls and now uses a wheelchair during the day. What is Violet's Waterlow score?

2   Early Warning Score (EWS): Simon Patrick has the following observations:

Respiratory rate	20 breaths per minute
SpO$_2$	95% on air
Blood pressure	120/74 mmHg
Heart rate	100 beats per minute
Neurological response	Alert

What is his EWS score?

3   A patient is prescribed 22 mg of gentamicin by injection. 20 mg in 2 mL of liquid for IM injection is available. How many millilitres will you administer?

4   A patient has been prescribed 30 mg of furosemide intravenously. 20 mg in 2 mL of liquid for IV injection is available. How many millilitres do you administer?

5   Diamorphine hydrochloride 10 mg is to be reconstituted in 10 mL of water for injection. A patient is prescribed a 20 mg bolus intramuscular injection. What volume of the drug needs to be administered?

NOTE: there is no displacement value to be considered.

6   Atenolol is available in a concentration of 5 mg in 10 mL. The patient is prescribed 2.5 mg IV as a bolus. It is to be given at a maximum rate of 1 mg/minute.

    (a) What volume of atenolol would you administer?

    (b) How many minutes should it be given over?

7   A patient is to receive 3 mg/mL of Adenocor, followed by a further 6 mg, then 12 mg, over a period of 6 minutes. What volume does the patient receive in total?

8   A morphine dose is calculated as 2 mg/kg for a concentrated solution.

    (a) A baby weighs 3.1 kg: how much morphine is prescribed to this infant?

    (b) The pump is running at 0.5 mL/hour. How many micrograms/kg per hour is the baby receiving?

9   500 mL of fluid is dripping at 35 drops per minute. The IV set delivers 15 drops/mL. How long will the infusion take?

10 Dopamine 150 mg is added to a bag of 500 mL of 5% dextrose. The prescription is to administer 6 micrograms/kg per minute of the infusate to a 75 kg patient. At what rate (in mL/hour) do you set the infusion pump?

KNOWLEDGE TEST 4

1   Malnutrition Universal Screening Tool (MUST): Sarah Hann is a 92-year-old lady who is 5 feet 4 inches in height and weighs 44 kg. What is her BMI?

2   Early Warning Score (EWS): Lesley David has the following observations:

Respiratory rate	10 breaths per minute
SpO_2	90% on air
Blood pressure	99/60 mmHg
Heart rate	51 beats per minute
Neurological response	Pain

What is his EWS score?

3   A patient has been prescribed 200 mg of co-amoxiclav. 600 mg in 10 mL of liquid for IV injection is available. How many millilitres do you administer?

4   Vancomycin is presented as a 1 g ampoule. It is to be diluted in 20 mL of water for injection. Your patient is prescribed 500 mg.

    (a)   What volume of vancomycin do you draw up? The vancomycin is to be added to a 500 mL bag of 0.9% saline. It is to be given at a rate of 4 mg/minute, due to the patient's fluid restriction.

    (b)   How many minutes must the infusion be given over?

    (c)   You are going to run it through an infusion pump. At what rate (in mL/hour) would you set the infusion pump?

5   A woman has been prescribed one unit of blood. The transfusion is to run over 3 hours. The unit consists of 350 mL of blood. The IV giving set (filtered) delivers 15 drops/mL. Calculate the drip rate in drops per minute.

6   Diamorphine hydrochloride 10 mg is to be reconstituted in 10 mL of water for injection. A patient is prescribed a 5 mg bolus intramuscular injection. What volume of the drug needs to be administered?

7   1000 mL of fluid is dripping at 20 drops per minute. The IV set delivers 15 drops/mL. How long will the infusion take?

8   Vancomycin is prescribed at 15 mg/kg BD. A baby patient weighs 975 g.

    (a)   What is the prescribed dose? Vancomycin comes as 500 mg in 10 mL. 1 mL is taken out (50 mg) and diluted 10 times to give a concentration of 50 mg in 10 mL. It is then infused over 1 hour.

    (b)   How much is going to be infused?

9 A patient weighing 65 kg is prescribed 500 micrograms/kg/h of aminophylline. 250 mg of aminophylline has been added to 100 mL of fluid.

    (a) How many mg/hour of aminophylline does the patient require?

    (b) At what rate (in millilitres per hour) would you set the infusion pump?

10 A patient weighing 70 kg has been prescribed 1.5 mg/kg of enoxaparin post-surgery. What amount do you administer?

Answers to Activity Questions

Activity 1.1

SECTION ONE
1 2.7
2 1.3
3 1.8
4 2.0
5 4.6

SECTION TWO
1 56
2 43
3 100
4 33
5 67

Activity 1.2

SECTION ONE
1 6 g
2 39 L
3 0.35 L
4 0.0007 mg
5 4 kg
6 4.5 g
7 800 micrograms
8 9000 ng
9 1.3 kg
10 0.000462 g

SECTION TWO
1 720 mg
2 1400 micrograms
3 30 mg
4 0.002 kg
5 2500 mL
6 700 micrograms
7 61 250 mL
8 92 000 g
9 20 micrograms
10 0.000023 g

SECTION THREE
1 0.02 mg
2 0.634 kg
3 63.5 micrograms
4 250 ng
5 8000 g
6 1.527 mg
7 21 900 mL
8 0.0645 mg
9 0.3498 kg
10 0.05 L

SECTION FOUR
1 3000 mL
2 1200 micrograms
3 40 micrograms
4 120 mg
5 0.00002 g

Calculation Skills for Nurses, First Edition. Claire Boyd
© 2013 John Wiley & Sons, Ltd. Published 2013 by John Wiley & Sons Ltd.

6 20 ng
7 2386 g
8 0.004 micrograms
9 1.234 L
10 0.32 g

Activity 1.3

1 90 mL
2 180 mL
3 80%
4 21.25%

Activity 1.4

1 8.3
2 7.5
3 35
4 20.8
5 41.7
6 17.4

Activity 1.5

1 (i) 25 mL (ii) 20 mL
2 (i) 566 mL (ii) 500 mL
3 (i) 55 mL (ii) 50 mL
4 (i) 200 mL (ii) 150 mL

Activity 1.6

1 19 + 19 + 19.5 + 18.0 + 17
= 82.5/5 = 18.5 mmHg

Activity 2.1

1 0.8
2 0.3
3 4.7
4 2.3
5 9.5
6 3.4
7 2.42
8 9.23

9 0.92
10 0.52
11 2.34
12 6.71
13 0.826
14 1.587
15 39
16 32
17 40

If you got any of questions **1–17** wrong, why not take a look at the Decimals section in Chapter 1.

18 6 g
19 0.00007 mg
20 9000 ng
21 30 mg
22 2500 mL
23 92 000 g
24 8000 g
25 0.0645 mg
26 1.527 mg
27 0.00002 g
28 1200 micrograms

If you got any of questions **18–28** wrong, why not take a look at the Metric Measures section in Chapter 1.

29 125 mL
30 61.3%
31 23.3%

If you got any of questions **29–31** wrong, why not take a look at the Percentages section in Chapter 1.

32 0.8
33 35.0
34 0.1

If you got any of questions **32–34** wrong, why not take a look at the Fractions section in Chapter 1.

35 1 in 5 = 1/5; 1/5 × 200 mL = 40 mL
36 1:5 = 1 in 6 = 1/6; 1/6 × 200 mL
= 33 mL to the nearest millilitre

37   1/3 × 600 mL = 200 mL
If you got any of questions **35–37** wrong, why not take a look at the Ratios section in Chapter 1.
38   19
39   4
40   60.48
If you got any of questions **38–40** wrong, why not take a look at the Averages section in Chapter 1.

Activity 3.1

1   3
2   38
3   0.25
4   0.00005
5   2
6   2.5
7   300
8   6000
9   1.6
10   0.000375
11   95.25 + 4.5 = 99.75
12   13 stone
13   400 micrograms = 0.4 mg; therefore the patient has taken 0.8 mg.
14   75 micrograms
15   0.935 kilograms
16   0.125 mg
17   1400 mL
18   0.027 grams
19   750 mg
20   7000 picograms

Activity 4.1a

1   2 tablets
2   ½ tablet
3   1½ tablets
4   The small amount needs to be converted into milligrams, which will result in even smaller amount. To change micrograms into milligrams, divide by 1000 (going up to the next decimal unit), giving 0.5 micrograms = 0.0005 mg. Then: $\frac{0.0005}{250} = 0.000002$ mg. This is not achievable but if this is the number you came up with then you are are correct.
5   ½ tablet
6   1½ tablets

Activity 4.1b

1   62.5 + 62.5 = 125.0 = 2 tablets
2   5 mg + 2 mg + 2 mg = 9 mg = 3 tablets
3 $\frac{300}{200} = 1.5 = 1½$ tablets
4   160 mg + 160 mg = 320 mg = 2 tablets
5   50 mg + 25 mg = 75 mg = 2 tablets
6 $\frac{250}{100} = 2.5 = 2½$ tablets

Activity 5.1

1 $\frac{50 \text{ mg}}{80 \text{ mg}} \times 2 \text{ mL} = 1.25 \text{ mL}$
2 $\frac{400 \text{ mg}}{500 \text{ mg}} \times 100 \text{ mL} = 80 \text{ mL}$
3 $\frac{20\,000 \text{ units}}{25\,000 \text{ units}} \times 1 \text{ mL} = 0.8 \text{ mL}$
4 $\frac{600 \text{ mg}}{400 \text{ mg}} \times 3 \text{ mL} = 4.5 \text{ mL}$
5   500 micrograms = 0.5 mg/0.5 mL + 500 micrograms = 0.5 mg/0.5 mL = 1 mg in 1 mL
6 $\frac{30 \text{ mg}}{20 \text{ mg}} \times 5 \text{ mL} = 7.5 \text{ mL}$
7   Change 1.2 grams into milligrams = 1200 mg

$\dfrac{800 \text{ mg}}{1200 \text{ mg}} \times 6 \text{ mL} = 3.9 \text{ mL}$

8 $\dfrac{250 \text{ mg}}{125 \text{ mg}} \times 5 \text{ mL} = 10 \text{ mL}$

9 $\dfrac{0.5 \text{ mg}}{0.6 \text{ mg}} \times 1 \text{ mL} = 0.83 \text{ mL}$

10 $\dfrac{1750 \text{ units}}{1000 \text{ units}} \times 1 \text{ mL} = 1.75 \text{ mL}$

Activity 6.1

1

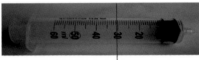

2

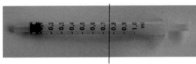

3 1.2 mL

Activity 6.2

Meniscus: approximately 29.0 mL

Activity 7.1

1 4 mL − 0.4 mL = 3.6 mL of water
2 Displacement value = 0.8 mL/1 g;
10 mL − 0.8 mL = 9.2 mL
3 Displacement value = 0.5 mL for
1 gram; 4 mL − 0.5 mL = 3.5 mL
4 Displacement value = 0.2 mL for
250 mg; 5 mL − 0.2 mL = 4.8 mL

Activity 8.1

1 70 kg × 10 mg = 700 mg
2 2.5 kg × 10 mg = 25 mg daily.
Divide this by 3 (to get 8-hourly
doses) = 8.33 mg, three times a day.

3 0.570 kg × 2 mg = 1.14 mg/day
4 148 kg × 30 mg = 1440 mg daily;
1440/3 = 480 mg/dose
5 15 kg × 40 mg = 600 mg daily;
600/4 = 150 mg/dose
6 20 kg × 80 mg = 1600 mg daily;
1600/4 = 400 mg/dose
7 58 kg × 100 mg = 5800 mg daily;
5800/4 = 1450 mg/dose
8 92 kg × 60 mg = 5520 mg daily;
5520/4 = 1380 mg/dose
9 35 kg × 20 mg = 700 mg daily;
700/3 = 233 mg/dose
10 20 kg × 45 mg = 900 mg daily;
900/4 = 225 mg/dose

Activity 9.1

1 First change 1.5 L into millilitres
= 1500 mL.
$\dfrac{1500}{12} \times \dfrac{20}{60} = 41.66 = 42$ drops
per minute (nearest whole drop).
2 $\dfrac{420}{4} \times \dfrac{15}{60} = 26.25 = 26$ drops
per minute
3 $\dfrac{150}{6} \times \dfrac{60}{60} = 25$ drops per minute
4 $\dfrac{350}{3} \times \dfrac{15}{60} = 29$ drops per minute
5 $\dfrac{500}{6} \times \dfrac{20}{60} = 27.77 = 28$ drops
per minute
6 (25 × 24 = 600) + (30 × 24 = 720)
= 1320 mL in 24 hours
7 $\dfrac{1000}{6} \times \dfrac{20}{60} = 55.55 = 56$ drops
per minute
8 $\dfrac{1500}{10} \times \dfrac{20}{60} = 50$ drops per minute
9 $\dfrac{260}{2} \times \dfrac{15}{60} = 32.5 = 33$ drops
per minute
10 $\dfrac{125}{1} \times \dfrac{15}{60} = 31.25 = 31$ drops
per minute
11 $\dfrac{200}{2} \times \dfrac{60}{60} = 100$ drops per minute
12 $\dfrac{150}{4} \times \dfrac{60}{60} = 37.5 = 38$ drops
per minute

Activity 10.1

1 Fluid left to infuse: 3000 mL
– 1500 mL = 1500 mL; hours left
to infuse: 24 – 8 = 16 hours
$\frac{1500}{16} \times \frac{20}{60} = 31.25 = 31$ drops
per minute

2 $\frac{600}{20} \times \frac{15}{60} = 7.5 = 7\frac{1}{2}$ hours

3 $\frac{1000}{20} \times \frac{15}{60} = 12.5 = 12\frac{1}{2}$ hours

4 Fluid left to infuse: 2000 mL
– 1500 mL = 500 mL; hours left to
infuse: 24 – 6 = 18 hours
$\frac{500}{18} \times \frac{20}{60} = 9.26 = 9$ drops
per minute

5 $\frac{1000}{43} \times \frac{20}{60} = 7\frac{3}{4}$ hours

Activity 11.1

1 $\frac{48 \text{ mL}}{24 \text{ hours}} = 2$ mL/hour

2 3 mL × 2 hours = 6.0 mL
3.5 mL × 3 hours = 10.5 mL
2 mL × 1 hour = 2.0 mL
2.5 mL × 1 hour = 2.5 mL
4 mL × 2 hours = 8.0 mL
29.0 units of Actrapid have been
received in total.

3 $\frac{1000 \text{ mL}}{8 \text{ hours}} = 125$ mL/hour

4 $\frac{500 \text{ mL}}{6 \text{ hours}} = 83.3$ mL/hour

5 $\frac{48 \text{ mL}}{12 \text{ hours}} = 4$ mL/hour

6 $\frac{1000 \text{ mL}}{12 \text{ hours}} = 83.3$ mL/hour

7 $\frac{24 \text{ mL}}{12 \text{ hours}} = 2$ mL/hour

8 $\frac{100 \text{ mL}}{0.5 \text{ hours}} = 200$ mL/hour
(remember: 30 mins = 0.5 hours)

9 $\frac{80 \text{ mL}}{0.5 \text{ hours}} = 160$ mL/hour

10 $\frac{75 \text{ mL} \times 60 \text{ minutes}}{20 \text{ minutes}} = 225$ mL/hour
(remember to convert the 75 mL
per minute into an hourly rate)

Activity 11.2

1 $\frac{50 \text{ mL} \times 60 \text{ minutes}}{20 \text{ minutes}}$
= 150 mL/hour

2 $\frac{100 \text{ mL} \times 60 \text{ minutes}}{30 \text{ minutes}}$
= 200 mL/hour

3 $\frac{100 \text{ mL} \times 60 \text{ minutes}}{30 \text{ minutes}}$
= 200 mL/hour

4 $\frac{120 \text{ mL} \times 60 \text{ minutes}}{50 \text{ minutes}}$
= 144 mL/hour

5 $\frac{80 \text{ mL} \times 60 \text{ minutes}}{50 \text{ minutes}}$
= 96 mL/hour

6 $\frac{60 \text{ mL} \times 60 \text{ minutes}}{45 \text{ minutes}} = 80$ mL/hour

Activity 11.3

(a) The cyclizine is available as
50 mg/1 mL, and the dose is
50 mg, so the volume to administer
would be 1 mL. Therefore 8 mL –
1 mL = 7 mL water for injection
if the cyclizine were to be
administered alone.

(b) 10 mg × 3 = 3 mL for the
diamorphine. Diamorphine 3 mL
+ cyclizine 1 mL = 4 mL in total
for the drugs; 8 mL – 4 mL for the
drugs = 4 mL of water for injection.

(c) 8 mL syringe = 48 mm;
$\frac{48 \text{ mm}}{24 \text{ hours}} = 2$ mm/hour

Activity 12.1

1 $\dfrac{50 \text{ mg}}{120 \text{ mg}} \times 5 \text{ mL} = 2.08 \text{ mL}$

2 $\dfrac{35 \text{ mg}}{15 \text{ mg}} \times 5 \text{ mL} = 11.66 \text{ mL}$

3 Weight × dose = 12 kg × 30 mg
   = 360 mg per daily dose/4 = 90 mg
   per single dose

4 Weight × dose = 36 kg × 80 mg
   = 2880 mg per daily dose/
   4 = 720 mg per single dose

5 2 stone 8 lb = (2 × 14) + 8 = 36
   pounds; 36 lb/2.2 kg = 16.36 kg

6 1 kg = 2.2 lb; 6.10 kg = 2.2 × 6.10
   = 13.42 lb; 1 lb = 16 oz = 0.42 lb
   × 16 oz = 6.72 oz. The baby
   weighs approximately 13 lb 7 oz.

7 **Step 1**: volume of all drugs per
   hour = 2 mL per hour + 8 mL every
   8 hours + 2 mL every 6 hours:
   8 mL/8 hours = 1 mL per hour;
   2 mL/6 hours = 0.33 mL every hour
   = 2 mL + 1 mL + 0.33 mL
   = 3.33 mL of the drug every hour.
   Step 2: $\frac{75}{100} \times 45 \text{ mL} = 33.75 \text{ mL}$
   = hourly fluid allowance
   Step 3: hourly fluid allowance
   minus the current drug volume
   = 33.75 mL − 3.33 mL = 30.42 mL
   Therefore, the total amount of
   feed that the child can receive is
   30.42 mL every hour.

8 Did you remember to convert the
   micrograms into milligrams, or
   milligrams into micrograms so that
   both units are the same?
   Change 125 micrograms into
   milligrams: 125/1000 = 0.125 mg
   $\dfrac{0.125 \text{ mg}}{0.5 \text{ mg}} \times 2 \text{ mL} = 0.5 \text{ mL}$

9 $\dfrac{20 \text{ mg}}{50 \text{ mg}} \times 1 \text{ mL} = 0.4 \text{ mL}$

10 BSA = approximately 0.72

11 BSA = approximately 0.69

12 $\dfrac{\text{Height} \times \text{weight}}{3600}$

   $= \dfrac{87 \text{ cm} \times 14.0 \text{ kg}}{3600} = 03383333$

   Square root = 0.58 m^2

Activity 13.1

1 6 × 150 mL = 900 mL; 900 + 188
   + 150 + 1500 mL = 2738 mL
   Fluid balance = 2738 − 750 mL
   = 1988 mL

Activity 13.2

1 Fluid balance: 1575 − 1110
   = 465 mL

2 Fluid balance: 1125 − 635 = 490 mL

3 Fluid balance: 950 − 900 = 50 mL

4 Fluid balance: 1750 − 500
   = 1250 mL

5 Fluid balance: 1150 − 100
   = 1050 mL

6 Fluid balance: 500 − 900
   = −400 mL (a negative amount)

Activity 14.1

Step 1 Obese, BMI = 31 kg/m^2, score = 0
Step 2 Score = 0
Step 3 Score = 2
Step 4 Total = 2, high risk
Step 5 Refer to dietician/nutritional
support; set goals; monitor and review.

Activity 15.1

1 EWS values: respiratory rate, 1;
   SpO$_2$, 1; blood pressure, 0; heart

rate, 0; neurological response (AVPU), 0; temperature, 0; total EWS, 2.

2 EWS values: respiratory rate, 2; SpO_2, 2; blood pressure, 0; heart rate, 3; neurological response (AVPU), 1; temperature, 1; total EWS, 9.

Activity 16.1

Waterlow scores: build, 3; skin type, 1; sex/age, 2 + 3; malnutrition, A = yes, B = 2; continence, 1; mobility, 3; special risks, tissue malnutrition, anaemia = 2; total Waterlow score, 17 (high risk).

Activity 17.1

1 2 tablets
2 4 tablets
3 1.5 mL. You need to be aware of speed shock.
4 ½ tablet
5 The dose is 1 mL, but you need to know when the patient last had this injection, as it is to be given once every 3 months.
6 3.5 mL. You need to be aware of speed shock.

Activity 17.2

1 ½ tablet
2 2½ tablets
3 ½ tablet
4 2 tablets
5 1½ tablets
6 1 tablet

Activity 18.1

1 Budget for education: £2200 per annum

Registered general nurses: venepuncture, 6 × £57.50 = £345; male catheterisation, 6 × £57.50 = £345
Care assistants: catheter care, 24 × £57.50 = £1380; Basic Clinical Skills 1 × £400 (12 staff) = £400
Total: £247; this exceeds the education budget by £270.00

2 6 registered general nurses:24 care assistants:12 customer services staff = 6:24:12 = 1:4:2

Activity 18.2

1 £119 billion
2 Social protection, £190 billion
3 £30 billion
4 £119 billion – £30 billion = £89 billion

Activity 19.1

1 Most hazards: acute transfusion reaction, ATR (34.8%).
2 Fewest hazards: post-transfusion purpura, PTP (0.1%).

Activity 19.2

Sodium: 145 mmol/L (133–146 mmol/L) = acceptable range
Bicarbonate: 30 mmol/L (22–29 mmol/L) = outside of acceptable range

Activity 20.1

1 $\dfrac{50 \text{ mg}}{80 \text{ mg}} \times 2 \text{ mL} = 1.25 \text{ mL}$

2 $\dfrac{300 \text{ mg}}{500 \text{ mg}} \times 100 \text{ mL} = 60 \text{ mL}$

3 $\dfrac{60 \text{ mg}}{30 \text{ mg}} = 2$ tablets

4 Weight × dose = 2.5 kg × 10 mg = 25 mg daily. Divide this by 3 to get the 8-hourly dose = 8.3 mg

5 $\dfrac{1000 \text{ mL}}{12 \text{ hours}} \times \dfrac{20 \text{ drops/mL}}{60 \text{ minutes}} = 27.77$
= 28 drops per minute (to nearest whole drop)

6 **(a)** $\dfrac{30\,000 \text{ units}}{25\,000 \text{ units}} \times 5 \text{ mL} = 6 \text{ mL}$

(b) Dilutant (48 mL) minus the volume of drug (6 mL) = 42.0 mL; this makes sure that we have a *total* of 48 mL in the syringe and not 48 *plus* 6 mL. This would make 54 mL, which is too much and a drug error.

7 $\dfrac{450 \text{ mL}}{4 \text{ hours}} \times \dfrac{15 \text{ drops/mL}}{60 \text{ minutes}} = 28.125$
= 28 drops per minute

8 $\dfrac{600 \text{ mL}}{20 \text{ drops per minute}}$
$\times \dfrac{15 \text{ drops/mL}}{60 \text{ minutes}} = 7.5 = 7\frac{1}{2}$ hours

9 $\dfrac{75 \text{ mg}}{100 \text{ mg}} \times 2 \text{ mL} = 1.5 \text{ mL}$

10 $\dfrac{225 \text{ mg}}{150 \text{ mg}} = 1.5 = 1\frac{1}{2}$ tablets

Activity 21.1

Patient A weighs 105 kg and has a height of 1.65 m. First, square the height 1.65 × 1.65 = 2.7225.
Next, divide the weight by the squared height:

$$105/2.7225 = 38.56$$
$$= 38.6 \text{ kg/m}^2$$

Therefore the patient falls into the obese category (BMI 30–39.9 kg/m^2).

Chapter 22
Knowledge test 1

1 Waterlow, Walter Jones: score = 13

2 EWS, Jane Fielding: respiratory rate, 0; SpO$_2$, 0; blood pressure, 0; heart rate, 0; neurological response (AVPU), alert 0; temperature, 0; total EWS, 0.

3 $\dfrac{35 \text{ mg}}{60 \text{ mg}} \times 1 \text{ mL} = 0.58 \text{ mL}$

4 $\dfrac{27 \text{ mg}}{30 \text{ mg}} \times 10 \text{ mL} = 9 \text{ mL}$

5 **(a)** Weight × dose = 100 kg × 10 mg = 1000 mg

(b) Change 4 g into milligrams = 4000 mg
$\dfrac{1000 \text{ mg}}{4000 \text{ mg}} \times 400 \text{ mL}$
= 100 mL/hour

6 **(a)** $\dfrac{15 \text{ mg}}{20 \text{ mg}} \times 2 \text{ mL} = 1.5 \text{ mL}$

(b) $\dfrac{15 \text{ mg}}{3 \text{ mg/min}} = 5$ minutes

7 $\dfrac{6 \text{ mg}}{15 \text{ mg}} \times 1 \text{ mL} = 0.4 \text{ mL}$

8 First change 1.5 g into milligrams = 1500 mg $\dfrac{1500 \text{ mg}}{500 \text{ mg}} \times 10 \text{ mL}$
= 30 mL

9 **(a)** Weight × dose = 1.2 kg × 2.5 mg = 3 mg

(b) $\dfrac{3 \text{ mg}}{5 \text{ mg}} \times 5 \text{ mL} = 3 \text{ mL}$
over 10 minutes

10 **(a)** Weight × dose = 3.4 kg × 50 mg = 170 mg

(b) $\dfrac{170 \text{ mg}}{600 \text{ mg}} \times 4 \text{ mL} = 1.13 \text{ mL}$

Knowledge test 2

1 MUST, Max Norman: 33 kg/m^2 = obese. Score on the MUST BMI chart = 0.

2 EWS, Robert Hayes: respiratory rate, 3; SpO$_2$, 2; blood pressure, 0; heart rate, 2; neurological response (AVPU), alert 0; temperature, 0; total EWS, 7.

3 $\dfrac{75 \text{ mg}}{50 \text{ mg}} \times 1 \text{ mL} = 1.5 \text{ mL}$

4 First change 75 micrograms into milligrams = 0.075 mg

$\dfrac{0.075 \text{ mg}}{0.1 \text{ mg}} \times 1 \text{ mL} = 0.75 \text{ mL}$

5 $\dfrac{275 \text{ micrograms}}{500 \text{ micrograms}} \times 2 \text{ mL} = 1.1 \text{ mL}$

6 First change 1 mg into micrograms = 1000 micrograms

$\dfrac{500 \text{ micrograms}}{1000 \text{ micrograms}} \times 1 \text{ mL} = 0.5 \text{ mL}$

7 Weight × dose = 90 kg × 80 mg = 7200 mg (daily dose)
Single dose (given 6 hourly):

$\dfrac{7200 \text{ mg}}{4} = 1800$ mg, or 1.8 grams

8 (a) Weight × dose = 4.2 kg × 50 mg/kg = 210 mg

(b) $\dfrac{210 \text{ mg}}{600 \text{ mg}} \times 4 \text{ mL} = 1.4 \text{ mL}$

9 **Step 1:** establish how much fluid left to infuse = 2000 mL − 700 mL = 1300 mL
Step 2: establish how much time is left to infuse = 24 hours − 10 hours = 14 hours
Step 3: $\dfrac{1300 \text{ mL}}{14 \text{ hours}} \times \dfrac{20 \text{ drops/mL}}{60 \text{ minutes}}$
= 30.9 = 31 drops per minute

10 3 mL × 1 hour = 3.0 mL
3.5 mL × 2 hours = 7.0 mL
2 mL × 2 hours = 4.0 mL
2.5 mL × 2 hours = 5.0 mL
4 mL × 1 hour = 4.0 mL
23.0 units of Actrapid have been received in total.

Knowledge test 3

1 Waterlow, Violet Simms: score = 20, high risk

2 EWS values, Simon Patrick: respiratory rate, 0; SpO$_2$, 0; blood pressure, 0; heart rate, 1; neurological response (AVPU), alert 0; temperature, 0; total EWS, 1.

3 $\dfrac{22 \text{ mg}}{20 \text{ mg}} \times 2 \text{ mL} = 2.2 \text{ mL}$

4 $\dfrac{30 \text{ mg}}{20 \text{ mg}} \times 2 \text{ mL} = 3 \text{ mL}$

5 $\dfrac{20 \text{ mg}}{10 \text{ mg}} \times 10 \text{ mL} = 20 \text{ mL}$

6 (a) $\dfrac{2.5 \text{ mg}}{5 \text{ mg}} \times 10 \text{ mL} = 5 \text{ mL}$

(b) $\dfrac{2.5 \text{ mg}}{1 \text{ mg/min}} = 2.5 \text{ minutes}$

7 3 mg is given in 1 mL, 6 mg in 2 mL and 12 mg in 4 mL
1 mL + 2 mL + 4 mL = total volume of 7 mL

8 (a) Weight × dose = 3.1 kg × 2 mg = 6.2 mg
Use this formula:

Dose (mg) × 1000 ÷ 50 ÷ weight (kg) × rate (mL/hour) = micrograms/kg per hour

(b) 6.2 × 1000 ÷ 50 ÷ 3.1 × 0.5 = 20 micrograms/kg per hour

9 $\dfrac{500 \text{ mL}}{35 \text{ drops/minute}} \times \dfrac{15 \text{ drops/mL}}{60 \text{ minutes}}$
$= 3.57 = $ just over 3½ hours

10 i 6 micrograms $= 0.006$ mg
$\times 60$ minutes $= 0.36$ mg/hour

ii Weight $\times$ dose $= 75$ kg $\times$
0.36 mg $= 27$ mg

iii $\dfrac{27 \text{ mg}}{150 \text{ mg}} \times 500 \text{ mL}$
$= 90$ mL/hour

Knowledge test 4

1 MUST, Sarah Hann: 17 kg/m^2.
Score on the MUST BMI chart $= 2$.

2 EWS values, Lesley David:
respiratory rate, 0; SpO$_2$, 1;
blood pressure, 1; heart rate, 0;
neurological response (AVPU),
pain 2; temperature, 0; total
EWS, 4.

3 $\dfrac{200 \text{ mg}}{600 \text{ mg}} \times 10 \text{ mL} = 3.33 \text{ mL}$

4 First change 1 g into milligrams
$= 1000$ mg

(a) $\dfrac{500 \text{ mg}}{1000 \text{ mg}} \times 20 \text{ mL} = 10 \text{ mL}$

(b) $\dfrac{500 \text{ mg}}{4 \text{ mg/min}} = 125$ minutes

(c) **Step 1:** add up total volume
of fluids $= 10$ mL vancomycin
$+ 500$ mL sodium chloride
$= 510$ mL

Step 2: change the rate per minute
into an hourly rate $= 4$ mg/minute
$\times 60$ minutes $= 240$ mg/hour

Step 3: $\dfrac{240 \text{ mg/hour}}{500 \text{ mg}} \times 510 \text{ mL}$
$= 244.8$ mL/hour

5 $\dfrac{350 \text{ mL}}{3 \text{ hours}} \times \dfrac{15 \text{ drops/mL}}{60 \text{ minutes}} = 29.16$
$= 29$ drops per minute

6 $\dfrac{5 \text{ mg}}{10 \text{ mg}} \times 10 \text{ mL} = 5 \text{ mL}$

7 $\dfrac{1000 \text{ mL}}{20 \text{ drops/minute}} \times \dfrac{15 \text{ drops/mL}}{60 \text{ minutes}}$
$= 12.5 = 12$½ hours

8 (a) First change grams into
kilograms $= 0.975$ kg
Weight $\times$ dose $= 0.975$ kg
$\times 15$ mg $= 14.625$ mg

(b) $\dfrac{14.625 \text{ mg}}{50 \text{ mg}} \times 10 \text{ mL}$
$= 2.925$ mL

9 (a) First change 500 micrograms
into milligrams $= 0.5$ mg
Weight $\times$ dose $= 65$ kg
$\times 0.5$ mg $= 32.5$ mg/hour

(b) $\dfrac{32.5 \text{ mg/hour}}{250 \text{ mg}} \times 100 \text{ mL}$
$= 13$ mL/hour

10 Weight $\times$ dose $= 70$ kg $\times 1.5$ mg
$= 105$ mg

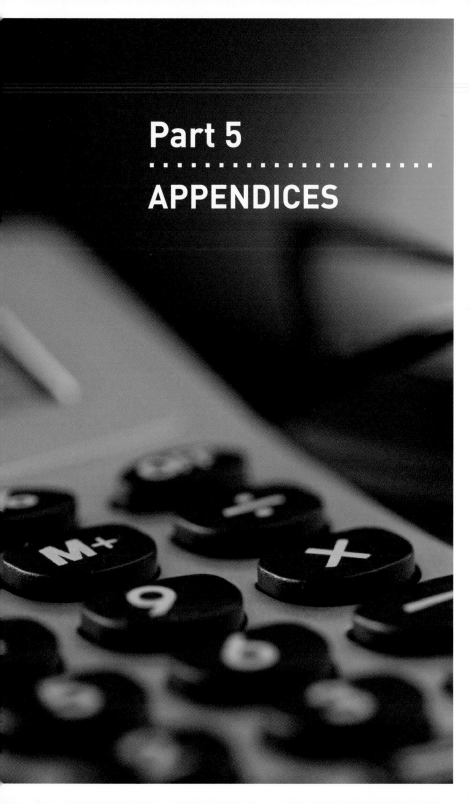

Part 5

APPENDICES

Appendix 1

FLUID CHART

Calculation Skills for Nurses, First Edition. Claire Boyd
2013 John Wiley & Sons, Ltd. Published 2013 by John Wiley & Sons Ltd.

FLUID CHART

24 h Fluid Record	NO:
	Surname:
Date: _____ . _____ . _____	Forenames:
Previous Day's Balance: _____mL	Dob:
	Ward:

Time	Input Route (mL)						Output Route (mL)				
Hour Ending	Oral	Enteral Tube				TOTAL	Urine	Gastric/ Vomit			TOTAL
08.00											
09.00											
10.00											
11.00											
12.00											
13.00											
14.00											
15.00											
16.00											
17.00											
18.00											
19.00											
20.00											
21.00											
22.00											
23.00											
24.00											
01.00											
02.00											
03.00											

Time	Input Route (mL)						Output Route (mL)				
Hour Ending	Oral	Enteral Tube				TOTAL	Urine	Gastric/ Vomit			TOTAL
04.00											
05.00											
06.00											
07.00											
24 h Total						24 h Input					24 h Input

24 h Balance =   mL

24 h Balance =   mL

Source: reproduced here with permission from North Bristol NHS Trust and University Hospitals Bristol NHS Foundation Trust.

Appendix 2

MALNUTRITION UNIVERSAL SCREENING TOOL

Calculation Skills for Nurses, First Edition. Claire Boyd
2013 John Wiley & Sons, Ltd. Published 2013 by John Wiley & Sons Ltd.

'Malnutrition Universal Screening Tool'

BAPEN
Advancing Clinical Nutrition

BAPEN is registered charity number 1023927   www.bapen.org.uk

'MUST'

'MUST' is a five-step screening tool to identify **adults,** who are malnourished, at risk of malnutrition (undernutrition), or obese. It also includes management guidelines which can be used to develop a care plan.

It is for use in hospitals, community and other care settings and can be used by all care workers.

This guide contains:

- A flow chart showing the 5 steps to use for screening and management
- BMI chart
- Weight loss tables
- Alternative measurements when BMI cannot be obtained by measuring weight and height.

The 5 'MUST' Steps

Step 1
Measure height and weight to get a BMI score using chart provided. *If unable to obtain height and weight, use the alternative procedures shown in this guide.*

Step 2
Note percentage unplanned weight loss and score using tables provided.

Step 3
Establish acute disease effect and score.

Step 4
Add scores from steps 1, 2 and 3 together to obtain overall risk of malnutrition.

Step 5
Use management guidelines and/or local policy to develop care plan.

Please refer to *The 'MUST' Explanatory Booklet* for more information when weight and height cannot be measured, and when screening patient groups in which extra care in interpretation is needed (e.g. those with fluid disturbances, plaster casts, amputations, critical illness and pregnant or lactating women). The booklet can also be used for training. See *The 'MUST' Report* for supporting evidence. Please note that 'MUST' has not been designed to detect deficiencies or excessive intakes of vitamins and minerals and is of **use only in adults.**

© BAPEN

Step 1 – BMI score (& BMI)

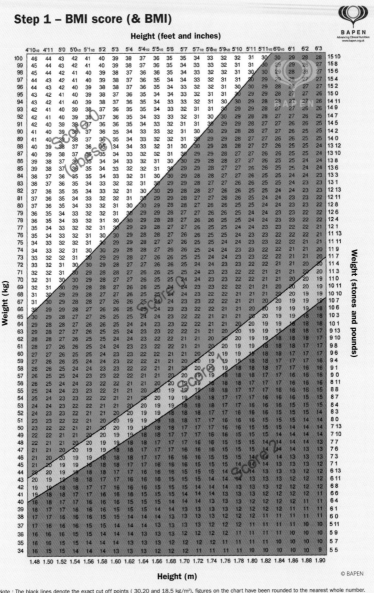

Note : The black lines denote the exact cut off points (30,20 and 18.5 kg/m²), figures on the chart have been rounded to the nearest whole number.

© BAPEN

Step 1
BMI score

+

Step 2
Weight loss score

+

Step 3
Acute disease effect score

BMI kg/m²	Score
>20 (>30 Obese)	= 0
18.5-20	= 1
<18.5	= 2

Unplanned weight loss in past 3-6 months

%	Score
<5	= 0
5-10	= 1
>10	= 2

If patient is acutely ill **and** there has been or is likely to be no nutritional intake for >5 days
Score 2

If unable to obtain height and weight, see reverse for alternative measurements and use of subjective criteria

Acute disease effect is unlikely to apply outside hospital. See 'MUST' Explanatory Booklet for further information

Step 4
Overall risk of malnutrition

Add Scores together to calculate overall risk of malnutrition
Score 0 Low Risk   Score 1 Medium Risk   Score 2 or more High Risk

Step 5
Management guidelines

0
Low Risk
Routine clinical care

- Repeat screening
  Hospital – weekly
  Care Homes – monthly
  Community – annually
  for special groups
  e.g. those >75 yrs

1
Medium Risk
Observe

- Document dietary intake for 3 days

- If adequate – little concern and repeat screening
  - Hospital – weekly
  - Care Home – at least monthly
  - Community – at least every 2-3 months

- If inadequate – clinical concern – follow local policy, set goals, improve and increase overall nutritional intake, monitor and review care plan regularly

2 or more
High Risk
Treat*

- Refer to dietitian, Nutritional Support Team or implement local policy

- Set goals, improve and increase overall nutritional intake

- Monitor and review care plan
  Hospital – weekly
  Care Home – monthly
  Community – monthly

* Unless detrimental or no benefit is expected from nutritional support e.g. imminent death.

All risk categories:

- Treat underlying condition and provide help and advice on food choices, eating and drinking when necessary.
- Record malnutrition risk category.
- Record need for special diets and follow local policy.

Obesity:

- Record presence of obesity. For those with underlying conditions, these are generally controlled before the treatment of obesity.

Re-assess subjects identified at risk as they move through care settings
See The 'MUST' Explanatory Booklet for further details and The 'MUST' Report for supporting evidence.

Step 2 – Weight loss score

BAPEN
Advancing Clinical Nutrition
www.bapen.org.uk

Weight before weight loss (kg)	SCORE 0 Wt Loss <5%	SCORE 1 Wt Loss 5-10%	SCORE 2 Wt Loss >10%
34 kg	<1.70	1.70 – 3.40	>3.40
36 kg	<1.80	1.80 – 3.60	>3.60
38 kg	<1.90	1.90 – 3.80	>3.80
40 kg	<2.00	2.00 – 4.00	>4.00
42 kg	<2.10	2.10 – 4.20	>4.20
44 kg	<2.20	2.20 – 4.40	>4.40
46 kg	<2.30	2.30 – 4.60	>4.60
48 kg	<2.40	2.40 – 4.80	>4.80
50 kg	<2.50	2.50 – 5.00	>5.00
52 kg	<2.60	2.60 – 5.20	>5.20
54 kg	<2.70	2.70 – 5.40	>5.40
56 kg	<2.80	2.80 – 5.60	>5.60
58 kg	<2.90	2.90 – 5.80	>5.80
60 kg	<3.00	3.00 – 6.00	>6.00
62 kg	<3.10	3.10 – 6.20	>6.20
64 kg	<3.20	3.20 – 6.40	>6.40
66 kg	<3.30	3.30 – 6.60	>6.60
68 kg	<3.40	3.40 – 6.80	>6.80
70 kg	<3.50	3.50 – 7.00	>7.00
72 kg	<3.60	3.60 – 7.20	>7.20
74 kg	<3.70	3.70 – 7.40	>7.40
76 kg	<3.80	3.80 – 7.60	>7.60
78 kg	<3.90	3.90 – 7.80	>7.80
80 kg	<4.00	4.00 – 8.00	>8.00
82 kg	<4.10	4.10 – 8.20	>8.20
84 kg	<4.20	4.20 – 8.40	>8.40
86 kg	<4.30	4.30 – 8.60	>8.60
88 kg	<4.40	4.40 – 8.80	>8.80
90 kg	<4.50	4.50 – 9.00	>9.00
92 kg	<4.60	4.60 – 9.20	>9.20
94 kg	<4.70	4.70 – 9.40	>9.40
96 kg	<4.80	4.80 – 9.60	>9.60
98 kg	<4.90	4.90 – 9.80	>9.80
100 kg	<5.00	5.00 – 10.00	>10.00
102 kg	<5.10	5.10 – 10.20	>10.20
104 kg	<5.20	5.20 – 10.40	>10.40
106 kg	<5.30	5.30 – 10.60	>10.60
108 kg	<5.40	5.40 – 10.80	>10.80
110 kg	<5.50	5.50 – 11.00	>11.00
112 kg	<5.60	5.60 – 11.20	>11.20
114 kg	<5.70	5.70 – 11.40	>11.40
116 kg	<5.80	5.80 – 11.60	>11.60
118 kg	<5.90	5.90 – 11.80	>11.80
120 kg	<6.00	6.00 – 12.00	>12.00
122 kg	<6.10	6.10 – 12.20	>12.20
124 kg	<6.20	6.20 – 12.40	>12.40
126 kg	<6.30	6.30 – 12.60	>12.60

Weight before weight loss (st lb)	SCORE 0 Wt Loss <5%	SCORE 1 Wt Loss 5-10%	SCORE 2 Wt Loss >10%
5st 4lb	<4lb	4lb – 7lb	>7lb
5st 7lb	<4lb	4lb – 8lb	>8lb
5st 11lb	<4lb	4lb – 8lb	>8lb
6st	<4lb	4lb – 8lb	>8lb
6st 4lb	<4lb	4lb – 9lb	>9lb
6st 7lb	<5lb	5lb – 9lb	>9lb
6st 11lb	<5lb	5lb – 10lb	>10lb
7st	<5lb	5lb – 10lb	>10lb
7st 4lb	<5lb	5lb – 10lb	>10lb
7st 7lb	<5lb	5lb – 11lb	>11lb
7st 11lb	<5lb	5lb – 11lb	>11lb
8st	<6lb	6lb – 11lb	>11lb
8st 4lb	<6lb	6lb – 12lb	>12lb
8st 7lb	<6lb	6lb – 12lb	>12lb
8st 11lb	<6lb	6lb – 12lb	>12lb
9st	<6lb	6lb – 13lb	>13lb
9st 4lb	<7lb	7lb – 13lb	>13lb
9st 7lb	<7lb	7lb – 13lb	>13lb
9st 11lb	<7lb	7lb – 1st 0lb	>1st 0lb
10st	<7lb	7lb – 1st 0lb	>1st 0lb
10st 4lb	<7lb	7lb – 1st 0lb	>1st 0lb
10st 7lb	<7lb	7lb – 1st 1lb	>1st 1lb
10st 11lb	<8lb	8lb – 1st 1lb	>1st 1lb
11st	<8lb	8lb – 1st 1lb	>1st 1lb
11st 4lb	<8lb	8lb – 1st 2lb	>1st 2lb
11st 7lb	<8lb	8lb – 1st 2lb	>1st 2lb
11st 11lb	<8lb	8lb – 1st 3lb	>1st 3lb
12st	<8lb	8lb – 1st 3lb	>1st 3lb
12st 4lb	<9lb	9lb – 1st 3lb	>1st 3lb
12st 7lb	<9lb	9lb – 1st 4lb	>1st 4lb
12st 11lb	<9lb	9lb – 1st 4lb	>1st 4lb
13st	<9lb	9lb – 1st 4lb	>1st 4lb
13st 4lb	<9lb	9lb – 1st 5lb	>1st 5lb
13st 7lb	<9lb	9lb – 1st 5lb	>1st 5lb
13st 11lb	<10lb	10lb – 1st 5lb	>1st 5lb
14st	<10lb	10lb – 1st 6lb	>1st 6lb
14st 4lb	<10lb	10lb – 1st 6lb	>1st 6lb
14st 7lb	<10lb	10lb – 1st 6lb	>1st 6lb
14st 11lb	<10lb	10lb – 1st 7lb	>1st 7lb
15st	<11lb	11lb – 1st 7lb	>1st 7lb
15st 4lb	<11lb	11lb – 1st 7lb	>1st 7lb
15st 7lb	<11lb	11lb – 1st 8lb	>1st 8lb
15st 11lb	<11lb	11lb – 1st 8lb	>1st 8lb
16st	<11lb	11lb – 1st 8lb	>1st 8lb
16st 4lb	<11lb	11lb – 1st 9lb	>1st 9lb
16st 7lb	<12lb	12lb – 1st 9lb	>1st 9lb

© BAPEN

Alternative measurements and considerations

BAPEN
Advancing Clinical Nutrition
www.bapen.org.uk

Step 1: BMI (body mass index)

If height cannot be measured
- Use recently documented or self-reported height (if reliable and realistic).
- If the subject does not know or is unable to report their height, use one of the alternative measurements to estimate height (ulna, knee height or demispan).

Step 2: Recent unplanned weight loss

If recent weight loss cannot be calculated, use self-reported weight loss (if reliable and realistic).

Subjective criteria

If height, weight or BMI cannot be obtained, the following criteria which relate to them can assist your professional judgement of the subject's nutritional risk category. Please note, these criteria should be used collectively not separately as alternatives to steps 1 and 2 of 'MUST' and are not designed to assign a score. Mid upper arm circumference (MUAC) may be used to estimate BMI category in order to support your overall impression of the subject's nutritional risk.

1. BMI
- Clinical impression – thin, acceptable weight, overweight. Obvious wasting (very thin) and obesity (very overweight) can also be noted.

2. Unplanned weight loss
- Clothes and/or jewellery have become loose fitting (weight loss).
- History of decreased food intake, reduced appetite or swallowing problems over 3-6 months and underlying disease or psycho-social/physical disabilities likely to cause weight loss.

3. Acute disease effect
- Acutely ill and no nutritional intake or likelihood of no intake for more than 5 days.

Further details on taking alternative measurements, special circumstances and subjective criteria can be found in *The 'MUST' Explanatory Booklet*. A copy can be downloaded at www.bapen.org.uk or purchased from the BAPEN office. The full evidence-base for 'MUST' is contained in *The 'MUST' Report* and is also available for purchase from the BAPEN office.

BAPEN Office, Secure Hold Business Centre, Studley Road, Redditch, Worcs, B98 7LG. Tel: 01527 457 850. Fax: 01527 458 718. bapen@sovereignconference.co.uk   BAPEN is registered charity number 1023927.   www.bapen.org.uk

Royal College of Nursing

Alternative measurements: instructions and tables

If height cannot be obtained, use length of forearm (ulna) to calculate height using tables below.
(See The 'MUST' Explanatory Booklet for details of other alternative measurements (knee height and demispan) that can also be used to estimate height).

Estimating height from ulna length

Measure between the point of the elbow (olecranon process) and the midpoint of the prominent bone of the wrist (styloid process) (left side if possible).

HEIGHT (m)														
Men (<65 years)	1.94	1.93	1.91	1.89	1.87	1.85	1.84	1.82	1.80	1.78	1.76	1.75	1.73	1.71
Men (≥65 years)	1.87	1.86	1.84	1.82	1.81	1.79	1.78	1.76	1.75	1.73	1.71	1.70	1.68	1.67
Ulna length (cm)	32.0	31.5	31.0	30.5	30.0	29.5	29.0	28.5	28.0	27.5	27.0	26.5	26.0	25.5
Women (<65 years)	1.84	1.83	1.81	1.80	1.79	1.77	1.76	1.75	1.73	1.72	1.70	1.69	1.68	1.66
Women (≥65 years)	1.84	1.83	1.81	1.79	1.78	1.76	1.75	1.73	1.71	1.70	1.68	1.66	1.65	1.63
Men (<65 years)	1.69	1.67	1.66	1.64	1.62	1.60	1.58	1.57	1.55	1.53	1.51	1.49	1.48	1.46
Men (≥65 years)	1.65	1.63	1.62	1.60	1.59	1.57	1.56	1.54	1.52	1.51	1.49	1.48	1.46	1.45
Ulna length (cm)	25.0	24.5	24.0	23.5	23.0	22.5	22.0	21.5	21.0	20.5	20.0	19.5	19.0	18.5
Women (<65 years)	1.65	1.63	1.62	1.61	1.59	1.58	1.56	1.55	1.54	1.52	1.51	1.50	1.48	1.47
Women (≥65 years)	1.61	1.60	1.58	1.56	1.55	1.53	1.52	1.50	1.48	1.47	1.45	1.44	1.42	1.40

Estimating BMI category from mid upper arm circumference (MUAC)

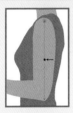

The subject's left arm should be bent at the elbow at a 90 degree angle, with the upper arm held parallel to the side of the body. Measure the distance between the bony protrusion on the shoulder (acromion) and the point of the elbow (olecranon process). Mark the mid-point.

Ask the subject to let arm hang loose and measure around the upper arm at the mid-point, making sure that the tape measure is snug but not tight.

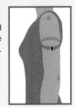

If MUAC is <23.5 cm, BMI is likely to be <20 kg/m^2.
If MUAC is >32.0 cm, BMI is likely to be >30 kg/m^2.

The use of MUAC provides a general indication of BMI and is not designed to generate an actual score for use with 'MUST'. For further information on use of MUAC please refer to *The 'MUST' Explanatory Booklet*.

© BAPEN

Source: the Malnutrition Universal Screening Tool (MUST) is reproduced here with the kind permission of BAPEN (British Association for Parenteral and Enteral Nutrition). For further information on MUST see www.bapen.org.uk.

Appendix 3

BRISTOL OBSERVATION CHART

Calculation Skills for Nurses, First Edition. Claire Boyd

2013 John Wiley & Sons, Ltd. Published 2013 by John Wiley & Sons Ltd.

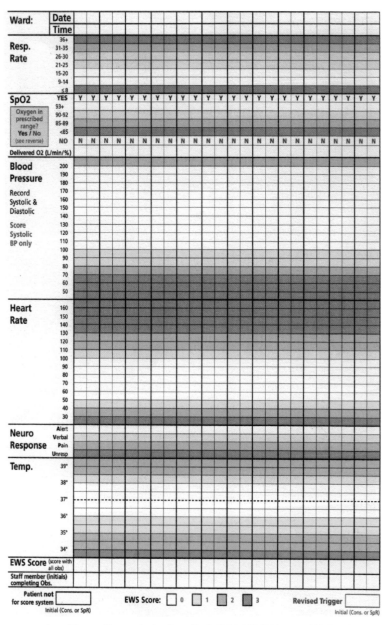

Source: reproduced here with permission from North Bristol NHS Trust and University Hospitals Bristol NHS Foundation Trust.

Appendix 4

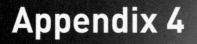

WATERLOW PRESSURE ULCER PREVENTION/ TREATMENT POLICY

Calculation Skills for Nurses, First Edition. Claire Boyd
2013 John Wiley & Sons, Ltd. Published 2013 by John Wiley & Sons Ltd.

(RING SCORES IN TABLE, ADD TOTAL: MORE THAN 1 SCORE/CATEGORY CAN BE USED)

BUILD/WEIGHT FOR HEIGHT ◆

Description	Score
AVERAGE — BMI (20–24.9)	0
ABOVE AVERAGE — BMI (25–29.9)	1
OBESE — BMI >30	2
BELOW AVERAGE — BMI >20	3

BMI = WT(kg)/ HT (m²)

SKIN TYPE VISUAL RISK AREAS ◆

Description	Score
HEALTHY	0
TISSUE PAPER	1
DRY	1
OEDEMATOUS	1
CLAMMY, PYREXIA	1
DISCOLOURED — STAGE 1	2
PRESSURE ULCER — STAGE 2–4	3

SEX/AGE ◆

Description	Score
MALE	1
FEMALE	2
14–49	1
50–64	2
65–74	3
75–80	4
81 +	5

NUTRITION ◆

A – HAS PATIENT LOST WEIGHT RECENTLY?
- YES – GO TO B
- NO – GO TO C
- UNSURE – GO TO C & SCORE 2

B – WEIGHT LOSS SCORE

Weight loss	Score
0.5–5kg	1
5–10kg	2
10–15kg	3
>15kg	4
UNSURE	2

C – PATIENT EATING POORLY/LACK OF APPETITE
- NO – SCORE 0   YES – SCORE 1

CONTINENCE ◆

Description	Score
COMPLETE/ CATHETERISED	0
URINE INCONT.	1
FAECAL INCONT.	2
URINARY + FAECAL INCONTINENCE	3

MOBILITY ◆

Description	Score
FULLY	0
RESTLESS/FIDGETY	1
APATHETIC	2
RESTRICTED	3
BEDBOUND e.g. TRACTION	4
CHAIRBOUND e.g. WHEELCHAIR	5

SPECIAL RISKS ◆

TISSUE MALNUTRITION ◆

Description	Score
TERMINAL CACHEXIA	8
MULTIPLE ORGAN FAILURE	8
SINGLE ORGAN FAILURE (RESP, RENAL, CARDIAC)	5
PERIPHERAL VASCULAR DISEASE	5
ANAEMIA (Hb < 8)	2
SMOKING	1

NEUROLOGICAL DEFICIT ◆

Description	Score
DIABETES, MS, CVA	4–6
MOTOR SENSORY	
PARAPLEGIA (MAX OF 6)	

MAJOR SURGERY OR TRAUMA ◆

Description	Score
ORTHOPAEDIC/SPINAL	5
ON TABLE > 2 HR*	5
ON TABLE > 6 HR*	8

MEDICATION

CYTOTOXICS, STEROIDS, ANTI-INFLAMMATORY MAX OF 4

SCORE	
10+	AT RISK
15+	HIGH RISK
20+	VERY HIGH RISK

Source: © Judy Waterlow 1985. Revised 2005.

Appendix 5

CONVERSION TABLES

Calculation Skills for Nurses, First Edition. Claire Boyd
2013 John Wiley & Sons, Ltd. Published 2013 by John Wiley & Sons Ltd.

KILOGRAMS TO POUNDS

1 kg = 2.2 lb

kg	lb	kg	lb	kg	lb	kg	lb	kg	lb	kg	lb
1	2.2	21	46.2	41	90.2	61	134.2	81	178.2	101	222.2
2	4.4	22	48.4	42	92.4	62	136.4	82	180.4	102	224.4
3	6.6	23	50.6	43	94.6	63	138.6	83	182.6	103	226.6
4	8.8	24	52.8	44	96.8	64	140.8	84	184.8	104	228.8
5	1.0	25	55.0	45	99.0	65	143.0	85	187.0	105	231.0
6	13.2	26	57.2	46	101.2	66	145.2	85	189.2	106	233.3
7	15.4	27	59.4	47	103.4	67	147.4	87	191.4	107	235.4
8	17.6	28	61.6	48	105.6	68	149.6	88	193.6	108	237.6
9	19.8	29	63.8	49	107.8	69	151.8	89	195.8	109	239.8
10	22.0	30	66.0	50	110.0	70	154.0	90	198.0	110	242.0
11	24.2	31	68.2	51	112.2	71	156.2	91	200.2	111	244.2
12	26.4	32	70.4	52	114.4	72	158.4	92	202.4	112	246.4
13	28.6	33	72.6	53	116.6	73	160.6	93	204.6	113	248.6
14	30.8	34	74.8	54	118.8	74	162.8	94	206.8	114	250.8
15	33.0	35	77.0	55	121.0	75	165.0	95	209.0	115	253.0
16	35.2	36	79.2	56	123.2	76	167.2	96	211.2	116	255.2
17	37.4	37	81.4	57	125.4	77	169.4	97	213.4	117	257.4
18	39.6	38	83.6	58	127.6	78	171.6	98	215.6	118	259.6
19	41.8	39	85.8	59	129.8	79	173.8	99	217.8	119	261.8
20	44.0	40	88.0	60	132.0	80	176.0	100	220.0	120	264.0

POUNDS TO KILOGRAMS

1 stone = 6.35 kg

stones	kg	stones	kg
1	6.35	15	95.25
2	12.7	16	101.6
3	19.05	17	107.95
4	25.4	18	114.3
5	31.75	19	120.65
6	38.1	20	127.0
7	44.45	21	133.35
8	50.8	22	139.7
9	57.15	23	146.05
10	63.5	24	152.4
11	69.85	25	158.75
12	76.2	26	165.1
13	82.55	27	171.45
14	88.9	28	177.8

STONES TO KILOGRAMS

1 lb = 0.45 kg

lb	kg
1	0.45
2	0.9
3	1.35
4	1.8
5	2.25
6	2.7
7	3.15
8	3.6
9	4.05
10	4.5
11	4.95
12	5.4
13	5.85
14 (1 stone)	6.35

Bibliography

Bolton-Maggs, P.H.B. (ed.) and Cohen, H. on behalf of the Serious Hazards of Transfusion (SHOT) Steering Group (2012) *The 2011 Annual SHOT Report.* www.shotuk.org/wp-content/uploads/2012/07/SHOT-ANNUAL-REPORT_FinalWebVersionBookmarked_2012_06_22.pdf.

British National Formulary (2009) *British National Formulary No. 58.* British Medical Association and Royal Pharmaceutical Society of Great Britain, London.

Davison, N. (2008) *Numeracy, Clinical Calculations and Basic Statistics: A Textbook for Healthcare Students.* Cromwell Press, Trowbridge.

Department of Education (1999) *The Moser Report.* HMSO, London.

Department of Health (2004) *Building a Safer NHS for Patients: Improving Medication Safety.* The Stationery Office, London.

Dougherty, L. and Lister, S. (eds) (2011) *The Royal Marsden Hospital Manual of Clinical Nursing Procedures,* 8th edn. Wiley-Blackwell, Oxford.

Downie, G., Mackenzie, J. and Williams, A. (2006) *Calculating Drug Doses Safely: A Handbook for Nurses and Midwives.* Churchill Livingstone, London.

Smith, J. and Roberts, R. (2011) *Vital Signs for Nurses – An Introduction to Clinical Observations.* Wiley-Blackwell, Oxford.

WEBSITES

www.bapen.org.uk
www.bbc.co.uk/skillswise/numbers
www.bddiabetes.com/us/hcp/main.asx
www.bnf.org/bnf/bnf/current/104945.htm
www.Judy.Waterlow.com.uk

Calculation Skills for Nurses, First Edition. Claire Boyd
© 2013 John Wiley & Sons, Ltd. Published 2013 by John Wiley & Sons Ltd.

Index

Calculation Skills for Nurses, First Edition. Claire Boyd
© 2013 John Wiley & Sons, Ltd. Published 2013 by John Wiley & Sons Ltd.

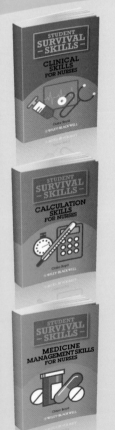
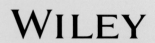